S T A T I S T I C S
P D Q

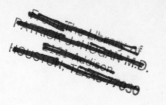

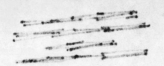

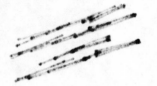

S**P**A**D**TIS**TI**C**Q**S

GEOFFREY R. NORMAN, Ph.D.

Associate Professor
Department of Clinical Epidemiology and Biostatistics
McMaster University Faculty of Medicine
Hamilton, Ontario

DAVID L. STREINER, Ph.D.

Professor of Psychiatry
Department of Clinical Epidemiology and Biostatistics
McMaster University Faculty of Medicine
Hamilton, Ontario

1986 B.C. Decker Inc • Toronto • Philadelphia

Publisher

B.C. Decker Inc.
3228 South Service Road
Burlington, Ontario   L7N 3H8

B.C. Decker Inc.
P.O. Box 30246
Philadelphia, Pennsylvania   19103

Sales and Distribution

United States and Possessions	**The C.V. Mosby Company** 11830 Westline Industrial Drive Saint Louis, Missouri 63146
Canada	**The C.V. Mosby Company, Ltd.** 5240 Finch Avenue East, Unit No. 1 Scarborough, Ontario M1S 4P2
United Kingdom, Europe and the Middle East	**Blackwell Scientific Publications, Ltd.** Osney Mead, Oxford OX2 OEL, England
Australia	**Holt-Saunders Pty. Limited** 9 Waltham Street Artarmon, N.S.W. 2064 Australia
Japan	**Igaku-Shoin Ltd.** Tokyo International P.O. Box 5063 1-28-36 Hongo, Bunkyo-ku, Tokyo 113, Japan
Asia	**Holt-Saunders Asia Limited** 10/F, Inter-Continental Plaza Tsim Sha Tsui East Kowloon, Hong Kong

PDQ Statistics   ISBN 0-941158-92-6

Library of Congress catalog card number: 86-71433

Printed in Singapore

10   9   8   7   6   5   4   3   2

To Pam, Betty, Adam, Leigh, Scott, Heather, and Shoshana

ACKNOWLEDGMENTS

We wish to acknowledge in particular the help we received from Pam Norman, who spent many hours with drafting pen in hand. Thanks also to the many secretaries and computer centre staff who reconfirmed the adage that computers are labor-saving devices that increase work.

CONTENTS

INTRODUCTION

WARNING: This is not an introductory textbook in statistics.

Introductory textbooks imply that you will go on to intermediate textbooks and then to advanced textbooks. As a result, introductory textbooks usually deal with only a few of the topics in the discipline. So if you want to apply your introductory knowledge of statistics to examining journals, most of the topics used by researchers won't have been covered.

Introductory textbooks have a couple of other problems. By and large they are written by experts with the hope of enticing others to become experts, so they are written in the language of the discipline. Now it is certainly an important goal to understand the jargon; in most cases once you get beyond the language things get a bit simpler. But jargon can be an impediment to learning. Also, beginning textbooks are usually written on the assumption that the only way you can understand an area is to plunge up to your neck in the nitty-gritty details of equation-solving, theorem-proving, or number-juggling. At some level that's probably legitimate. We're not sure we'd like a surgeon to remove an appendix who has a good conceptual grasp of the relevant anatomy and operating procedures, but who hasn't actually done it. But we are going to assume that all that work is not necessary to understand an area, so we'll try to minimize the use of algebra, calculus, and calculations, and we'll use ordinary English as much as possible.

The intent of this book is to help you through the Results section of the research article where the numbers are actually crunched, and little asterisks or "$P < 0.05$" values appear as if by magic in the margins, to the apparent delight of the authors. We think that by reading this book, you won't actually be able to *do* any statistics (actually, with computers on every street corner, no one— doctor, lawyer, beggarman, or statistician—should have to do statistics), but you will understand what researchers are doing, and may even be able to tell when they're doing it wrong. There is an old joke about the three little French boys, aged four, five, and six who saw a man and a women naked on a bed in a basement apartment. They said:

Four Year Old: Look at that man and that women in there! They are wrestling!

Five Year Old: No silly, they are making love.

Six Year Old : Yes, and very poorly too!

The four year old knew nothing of lovemaking. The five year old had achieved a conceptual understanding, and the six year old understood lovemaking sufficiently well, presumably without having actually done it, to be a critical observer. The challenge of this book will be to turn you into a six year old statistician. So, we will not take the "Introductory Textbook" approach in this book. Instead, we will expose you to nearly every kind of statistical method you are likely to encounter in your reading. Our aim will be to help you understand what is going on with a particular approach to analysis, and furthermore, we hope you will understand enough to recognize when the author is using the method incorrectly. Along the way, you can leave the calculator on the back shelf, because it won't be needed. One cautionary note. It would be nice if we could hand you an encyclopedia of statistical tests so you could just turn to page whatever and read about the particular test of interest. But statistics isn't quite like that. Like most things in science, it is built up logically on fundamental principles and evolves gradually to greater complexity. In order to gain some appreciation of the underlying concepts, it probably behooves you to start at the beginning and read to the end of the book at least once.

We hope that as a result of reading the book you will find the results section of journal articles a little less obscure and intimidating and thereby become a more critical consumer of the literature. It would not be surprising if you emerged with a certain degree of skepticism as a result of your reading. However, it would be unfortunate if you ended up dismissing out of hand any research using advanced statistical methods simply because of your knowledge of the potential pitfalls. Keep in mind that the objective of all statistical analysis is to reveal underlying systematic variation in a set of data, either as a result of some experimental manipulation or from the effect of other measured variables. The strategy, which forms the basis of all statistical tests, is a comparison between an observed effect or difference and the anticipated result of random variation. Like a good stereo receiver, statistical analysis is designed to pluck a faint signal out of a sea of noise.

Unfortunately, also like a modern stereo receiver, the statistical methods are contained in black boxes like BMDP, SPSS-X, or Minitab; prominent stickers proclaim that they should be opened by qualified personnel only so that it is nearly impossible to understand the detailed workings of a MANOVA, factor analysis, or logistic regression program. Finally, to complete the analogy, these boxes of software seem replete with endless switches and dials in the form of obscure tests or optional approaches, which may be selected in order to execute the programs and report the results.

It is understandable that many people in the research community react toward new statistical methods in the same way that they might react to other new technology; either they embrace the techniques openly and uncritically, or they reject any examples out of hand. Neither response is appropriate. These methods, available now through the development of sophisticated computer hardware and software, have made an enormous contribution to research in the social and health sciences. Nevertheless, they can be used appropriately or they can be abused, and the challenge that faces the reader is to decide whether a particular example is one or the other.

Let us say ahead of time what statistics cannot do in order to place the book in an appropriate context.

The probability or "p" level associated with any test of significance is only a statement of the likelihood that an observed difference could have arisen by chance. Of itself, it says nothing about the size or importance of an effect. Because probability level is so closely related to sample size, small effects in large studies can achieve impressive levels of significance. Conversely, studies involving small numbers of subjects may have too little power to detect even fairly large effects.

No statistical method can effectively deal with the systematic biases that may result from a poorly designed study. For example, statistical techniques may be used to adjust for initial differences between two groups, but there is no way to ensure that this adjustment compensates exactly for the effect of these differences on the results of the study. Similarly, no statistical analysis can compensate for low response rates or high dropouts from a study. We can demonstrate *ad nauseam* that the subjects who dropped out had the same age, sex, marital status, education, and income as those who stayed in, but this is no guarantee that they would have been comparable on the variables that were measured in the study. The mere fact that they dropped out implies that they were different on at least one dimension, namely the inclination to remain in the study. Finally, no measure of association derived from natural variation in a set of variables, however strong, can establish with certainty that one variable *caused* another. To provide you with some tools to sort out the different experimental designs, we have included a critical review of the strengths and weaknesses of several designs in Chapter 18.

Finally, even after you are satisfied that a study was conducted with the appropriate attention to experimental design and statistical analysis and that the results are important, there remains one further analysis which you, the reader, can conduct. Whether you are a researcher or clinician, you must examine whether the results are applicable to the people with whom you deal. Are the people studied in the research paper sufficiently similar to your patients that the effects or associations are likely to be similar? For example, treatments that have significant effects when applied to severely ill patients in a university teaching hospital may be ineffective when used to treat patients with the same, albeit milder form of the disease, that is encountered in a general practice. Similarly, psychological tests developed on university undergraduates may yield very different results when applied to a middle-aged general population. The judgment as to the applicability of the research results to your setting rests primarily on the exercise of common sense and reasoning, nothing more.

One last word about the intent of this book. Although we would like to think that a good dose of common sense and an understanding of the concepts of statistics will enable you to examine the literature critically, we're going to hedge our bets a bit. Throughout the book we will highlight particular areas where researchers frequently misuse or misinterpret statistical tests. These will be labelled as "C.R.A.P.* Detectors", with apologies to Ernest Hemingway,** and are intended to provide particular guides for you to use in reviewing any study.

---

* Circular Reasoning or Anti-intellectual Pomposity
** Postman, Weingartner. Teaching as a subversive activity.

In applying your new knowledge, don't be intimidated by all the tables of numbers and hifalutin talk. Always keep in mind the advice of Winifred Castle, a British statistician, who wrote that "We researchers use statistics the way a drunkard uses a lamp post, more for support than illumination". Finally, we hope that you enjoy the book!

G. R. N.
D. L. S.
May, 1986

VARIABLES AND DESCRIPTIVE STATISTICS

NAMES AND NUMBERS: TYPES OF VARIABLES

> There are four types of variables. *Nominal* and *ordinal* variables consist of counts in categories and must be analysed using "non-parametric" statistics. *Interval* and *ratio* variables are actual quantitative measurements and are analysed using "parametric" methods.

Statistics provide a way of dealing with numbers. Before leaping headlong into statistical tests, it is necessary to get some idea of how these numbers come about, what they represent, and the various forms the numbers can take.

Let's begin by examining a simple experiment. Suppose an investigator has a hunch that clam juice is an effective treatment for the misery of psoriasis. He proceeds to assemble a group of patients, randomizes them to a treatment and control group and gives clam juice to his treatment group and something which looks, smells and tastes like clam juice, but isn't, to his control group. After a few weeks, he measures the extent of psoriasis on the patients, perhaps by estimating the percent of the body involvement, or by looking at the change in size of a particular lesion. He then proceeds to do some number-crunching to determine if clam juice is as good as he hopes it is.

Let's have a closer look at the data from this experiment. To begin with, there are at least two variables. A definition of the term variable is a little hard to come up with, but basically it relates to anything which is measured or manipulated in the study. The most obvious variable in the experiment is the measurement of the extent of psoriasis. It is pretty evident that this is something which can be measured. A less obvious variable is the nature of treatment—drug or placebo. Although it is less evident how you might convert this to a number, still it is clearly something which is varied in the course of the experiment.

A few more definitions are in order. We frequently speak of independent and dependent variables. In an experiment, the independent variables are those which are varied by, and under the control of, the experimenter, and the dependent variables are those which respond to the experimental manipulation. In the present example, the independent variable is the type of therapy—clam juice or placebo—and the dependent variable is the size of lesions or body involvement. Although in this example the identification of independent and dependent variables is straightforward, the distinction is not always so obvious. Frequently researchers must rely on natural variation in both types of variables and look for a relationship between the two. For example, in looking for a relation between smoking and lung cancer, an ethics committee would probably take a dim view of ordering a thousand children to smoke a pack a day for 20 years. Instead, the investigator must simply look for a relationship between smoking and cancer in the general population and assume smoking is the independent variable and lung cancer is the dependent variable; that is, the extent of lung cancer *depends* on variations in smoking.

There are other ways of defining types of variables which turn out to be essential in determining the ways the numbers will be analyzed. Variables are frequently classified as nominal, ordinal, interval, or ratio. A nominal variable is simply a *named* category. Our clam juice vs. placebo is one such variable, as is the sex of the patient, or the diagnosis given to a group of patients.

An ordinal variable is a set of *ordered* categories. A common example in the medical literature is the subjective judgment of disease staging in cancer, using categories such as stage I, II, or III. Although we can safely say that stage II is worse than stage I, and better than stage III, we don't really know by how much.

The other kinds of variables consist of actual measurements on individuals, such as height, weight, blood pressure, or serum electrolytes. Statisticians distinguish between interval variables, where the interval between measurements is meaningful (e.g., 38° − 32° Celsius), and ratio variables, where the ratio of the numbers has some meaning. Having made the distinction, they then go and analyse them all the same anyway. The important distinction is that these variables are measured *quantities*, unlike nominal and ordinal variables that are *qualitative* in nature.

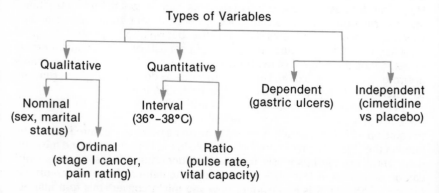

Figure 1.1   Types of variables

So where does the classification lead us? The important distinction is between the nominal and ordinal variables on one hand, and the interval and ratio variables on the other. It makes no sense to speak of the average value of a nominal or ordinal variable—the average sex of a sample of patients or, strictly speaking, the average disability expressed on an ordinal scale. However, it is sensible to speak of the average blood pressure or average height of a sample of patients. For nominal variables, all we can really deal with is the number of patients in each category. Statistical methods applied to these two broad classes of data are very different. For measured variables, it is generally assumed that the data follow a bell curve and that the statistics focus on the center and width of the curve. These are the so-called parametric statistics. By contrast, nominal and ordinal data consist of counts of people or things in different categories, and a different class of statistics, called non-parametric statistics (obviously!) is used in dealing with these data.

Example 1.1

To examine a program for educating health professionals in a sports injury clinic about the importance of keeping detailed records, a researcher does a controlled trial in which the *dependent* variable is range of motion of injured joints, which is classified as (a) worse, (b) same, or (c) better, and the *independent* variable is (a) program or (b) no program.

Question

What kind of variables are they—nominal or ordinal? Are they appropriate?

Answer

The independent variable is *nominal*, and the dependent variable, as stated, is *ordinal*. However, there are two problems with the choice. First, detailed medical records may be a good thing and may even save some lives somewhere. But range of motion is unlikely to be sensitive to changes in recording behavior. A better choice would be some rating of record quality. Second, range of motion is a nice ratio variable. To shove it into three categories is just throwing away information.

C.R.A.P. Detector #1.1

Dependent variables should be sensible. Ideally, they should be clinically important, but also related to the independent variable.

C.R.A.P. Detector #1.2

In general, the amount of information increases as one goes from nominal to ratio. Classifying good ratio measures into large categories is akin to throwing away data.

DESCRIBING DATA
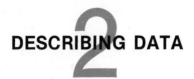

A key concept in statistics is the use of a frequency distribution to reflect the probability of occurrence of an event. The distribution can be characterized by measures of the average—mean, median, and mode, and measures of dispersion—range and standard deviation.

Once a researcher has completed a study, he is faced with a major challenge: to analyze his data so he can publish, add a line on his résumé, get promoted or tenured, get more research grants, analyze more data.

There are two distinct steps in the process of analyzing the data. The first is to describe the data, using standard methods to determine the average value, the range of data around the average, and other characteristics. The objective of descriptive statistics is simply to communicate the results without attempting to generalize beyond the sample of individuals to any other group. This is an important first step in any analysis. For the reader to understand the basis for the conclusions of any study, he must have some idea of what the data look like.

The second step in some, but not all, studies is to infer the likelihood that the observed results can be generalized to other samples of individuals. If we want to show that clam juice is an effective treatment for psoriasis or that IQ is related to subsequent performance, we are attempting to make a general statement that goes beyond the particular individuals we have studied. The rub is that differences between groups can rarely be attributed simply to the experimental intervention: some people in the clam juice group may get worse, and some people in the placebo group may get better. The goal of inferential statistics is to determine the likelihood that these differences could have occurred by chance, as a result of the combined effects of unforseen variables not under direct control of the experimenter. It is here the statistical heavy artillery is brought to bear. As a result, most damage to readers of journals is inflicted by inferential statistics. Most of this book is devoted to the methods of statistical inference. But a good idea of what the data look like is a necessary prerequisite to complex statistical analysis, both for the experimenter and the reader, so let's start there.

FREQUENCIES AND DISTRIBUTIONS

Whether a study involves 10 or 10,000 subjects, eventually the researcher ends up with a collection of numbers, often glorified by such names as "data set" or "data base." In the case of nominal or ordinal variables, the numbers are some indicator of the category to which each subject belongs (e.g., the sex, religion, or the diagnosis of each subject). For interval and ratio variables, the researcher will have the actual numerical value of the variable for each subject—the subject's height, blood pressure, pulse rate, or number of cigarettes smoked. There is a subtle difference among these latter variables, by the way, even though all are ratio variables. Things like height and blood pressure are continuous variables: they can be measured to as many decimal places as the measuring instrument allows. By contrast, although the average American family has 2.1 children, no one has ever found the family with one-tenth of a child, and counts such as this are discrete variables.

In either case, these numbers are distributed in some manner among the various categories or over the various possible values. If you were to plot the numbers, you would end up with distributions similar to Figures 2.1 and 2.2.

Note that there are a couple of things that can be done to make these figures more understandable. If we simply divide the numbers in each category by the total number of people studied, we are then displaying the proportion of the total sample in each category, as shown on the right side of the graph. Some manipulations can be performed on these proportions; for example, to find the

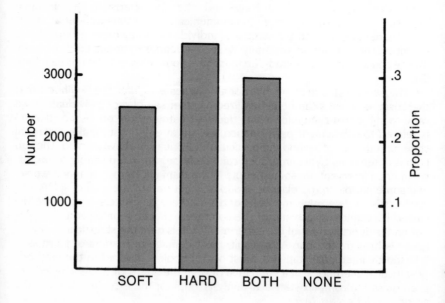

Figure 2.1   Distribution of ice cream preferences in 10,000 school children

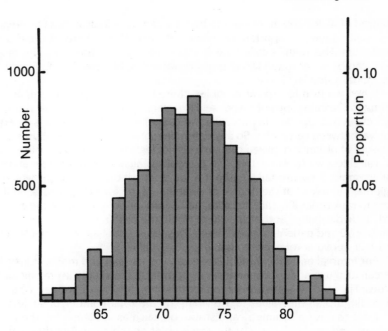

Figure 2.2   Age distribution of 10,000 entrants in senior citizen roller derby

probability in Figure 2.2 that one of our folks is 69 or 70 years old, we must add up the probabilities in these two year categories. We can also address questions such as, "What is the probability that a senior citizen is over 71 years of age?" by adding up the categories above age 71 years.

The basic notion is that we can view the original distribution of numbers as an expression of the probability that any individual chosen at random from the original sample may fall in a particular category, or within a range of categories. This transformation from an original frequency distribution to a distribution of probability is a recurrent and fundamental notion in statistics.

Although a frequency distribution is a convenient way to summarize data, it has certain disadvantages. It is difficult to compare two distributions derived from different samples because the information is buried in the number of responses in each category. It's also tedious to draw graphs and a lot easier to get the computer to blurt out a series of numbers. As a result, some way to summarize the information is necessary. The conventional approach is to develop standard methods to describe where the center of the distribution lies, and how wide it is.

MEANS, MEDIANS, AND MODES: MEASURES OF THE MIDDLE

For nominal data, there is no ordering implied in the various categories; we can't say that a preference for hard ice cream is, in any sense, better than a hatred of all ice cream. About the best we can do is indicate which category was most frequently reported, i.e., in our ice cream study "hard" was indicated most often. This value is called the modal value of the distribution. This modal value can be determined for all types of variables. For example, in Figure 2.2 the modal value is 73.

When we turn to ordinal variables, there is now an explicit or implied ordering to the categories of response. However, we don't really know the spacing between categories. In particular, we cannot assume that there is an equal interval between categories. So any determination of an average that uses some measure of distance between categories is not legitimate. However, unlike nominal variables, we do know that one category is higher or lower than another. For example, if we are talking about a rating of patient disability, it would be legitimate to ask what the degree of disability of the average *patient* is. So if we were to rank order 100 patients, with the "no disability" patients at the bottom, and "total disability" at the top, where would the dividing line between patient number 50 and patient number 51 be? This value, with half the subjects below and half above is referred to as the median value.

For interval and ratio variables, we can use median and modal values, but we can also use a more commonsense approach, i.e., simply averaging all the values. The mean is statistical jargon for this straightforward average, obtained by adding up all the values and dividing by the total number of subjects.

Note that for a symmetrical distribution, such as in Figure 2.2, the mean, median, and mode all occur at the same point on the curve. But this is not always the case; for example, if we were to plot the distribution of income of physicians, it might look like Figure 2.3.

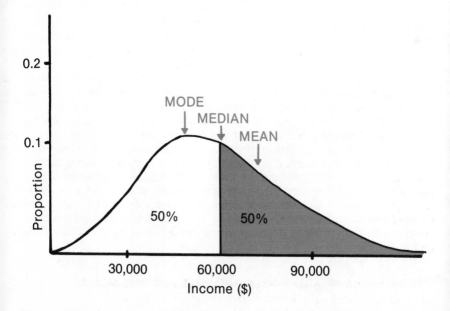

Figure 2.3   Distribution of physician income

The *modal* value, the high point of the curve, would be at about $50,000, the *median* income of the doc at the 50th percentile would be about $60,000, and the few rich specialists may push the *mean* or average income up to around $70,000. (Admittedly, these numbers are woefully behind the times.) This kind of curve is referred to as a "skewed" distribution, in this particular case positively skewed. In general, if the curve has one tail longer than the other, the mean is always toward the long tail, the mode nearer the short tail, and the median somewhere between the two.

As a final wrinkle, in some data there may be two or more high points in the distribution such as is shown in Figure 2.4. In this case, the distribution has two modes, love and hate, and is referred to as "bimodal."

MEASURES OF VARIATION: RANGE, PERCENTILE, STANDARD DEVIATION

The various ways of determining an average provide a first step in the development of summary measures of distributions, but we also need some measure of the extent to which individual values differ from the mean. The most obvious measure of dispersion is the range. For nominal variables, since the categories are not ordered, the range is simply the number of categories with at least one response. For the other variables, the range is the difference between the highest and lowest values.

For ordinal, interval, and ratio variables there is another way to think about variation which is a natural extension of concept of the median. As you will recall, the median was defined as the point where 50 percent of the sample were below, and 50 percent above, that value. The locations of the 0th and 100th per-

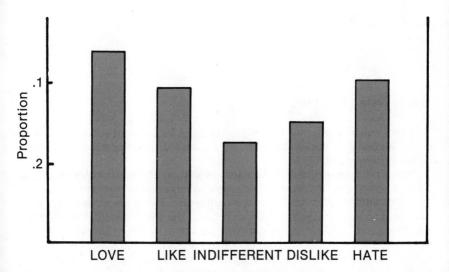

Figure 2.4   Distribution of attitudes to parents of 100 teenagers

centile would define the range. More commonly, people define the value of the 5th and 95th percentile, with 5 percent of people below, and 95 percent of people below, as some measure of dispersion. In the same vein, the distribution can be divided into "quartiles" using cutpoints at 25 percent, 50 percent, and 75 percent; thus, the "interquartile range" is the difference between the values of the 25th and 75th percentile.

For interval and ratio variables, there is another approach to measuring the dispersion of individual values about the mean that bears the name "average deviation." To compute the average deviation, first calculate the difference between each datum and the mean, then sum all the differences, and divide by the number of data points. The only problem is that there are as many negative differences from the mean as positive differences, and a little algebra will show that the average deviation calculated this way always turns out to be zero.

A simple way around the problem of negative differences is to square each term (multiply it by itself) so that all the terms are positive. You then would have terms such as: (individual value − mean value)^2. If all these terms are summed, and the total is then divided by the number of terms, the result is an average squared deviation and is called a variance. Well and good, except that variances are no longer in the same unit of measurement as the original data. For example, if height were measured in inches, the units of variance would be square inches. So the final step is to take the square root of this quantity, resulting in the standard measure of dispersion called the standard deviation. The standard deviation, then, is a slightly devious way of determining, on the average, how much individual values differ from the mean. The smaller the standard deviation (S.D., or s), the less each score varies from the mean. The larger the spread of scores, the larger the standard deviation becomes. Algebraically, the formula looks like this:

$$\text{Standard Deviation} = \sqrt{\frac{\text{Sum of (Individual Value} - \text{Mean)}^2}{\text{Number of Values}}}$$

THE NORMAL DISTRIBUTION

Since much of what we will be discussing in subsequent sections is based on the normal distribution, it's probably worthwhile spending a little more time showing where it all fits in.

It has been observed that the natural variation of many variables tends to follow a bell-shaped distribution, with most values clustered symmetrically near the mean and a few values falling out on the tails. The shape of this bell curve can be expressed mathematically in terms of the two statistical concepts we have discussed—the mean and standard deviation. In other words, if you know the mean and S.D. of your data, and if you are justified in assuming the data follow a normal distribution, then you can tell precisely the shape of the curve by plugging the mean and standard deviation into the formula for the normal curve.

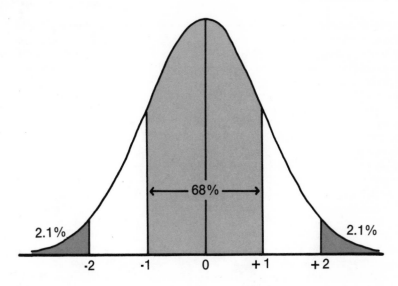

Figure 2.5   The normal distribution

If you then look at the calculated curve superimposed on your mean and standard deviation, it would look something like Figure 2.5.

Sixty-eight percent of the values fall within one standard deviation of the mean, 95 percent within two standard deviations and 2.5 percent in each tail. This is true for every normal distribution, not just this curve, and comes from the theoretical shape of the curve. This is a good thing because our original figures, such as those in Figure 2.2, don't really give much idea of what is happening out on the tails. But we can use all the data to get a good estimate of the mean and standard deviation, then draw a nice smooth curve through it.

That just about completes our Cook's tour of descriptive statistics. We have not attempted to show you all the ways data can be displayed, nor have we indicated the devious ways to distort the truth with graphs and figures. A little book called *How to Lie with Statistics*[*] has an excellent discussion of ways people distort data to suit their own ends and has far more useful C.R.A.P. detectors for consumers of descriptive data than we could offer in this brief chapter. The important point, which we raised in the previous chapter, is simply that the onus is on the author to convey to the reader an accurate impression of what his data look like, using graphs or standard measures, before he starts the statistical shenanigans. Any paper which doesn't do this should be viewed from the outset with considerable suspicion.

---

[*] Darrell Huff. ''How to lie with statistics''. New York: Penguin Books, 1954.

PARAMETRIC STATISTICS

STATISTICAL 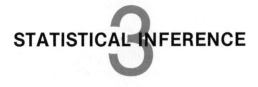 INFERENCE

> Statistical inference is the process of inferring features of the population from observations of a sample. The analysis addresses the question of the likelihood that an observed difference could have arisen by chance. The "z" test is the simplest example of a statistical test and examines the difference between a sample and a population, when the variable is a measured quantity.

The story goes that one day Isaac Newton was slacking off in an apple orchard when an apple fell on his head and he invented the law of gravitation. It's a pretty safe bet that Newton's goal wasn't really to describe the motion of apples falling off trees—they don't usually hand out Nobel prizes for things like that. Rather, he was attempting, successfully as it turns out, to formulate a general rule based on his observations of specific instances.

Forgive a moment's pomposity, but that is really what science is all about: to derive general rules that describe a large class of events, as a result of observation and experiment of a limited subset of this class. There are at least two issues in this generalization. The first is that if the scientist wishes to have confidence in his generalization, he must be fairly sure that the people or things he chooses to study are representative of the class he wants to describe. This is a notion that leads to the fundamental role of random sampling in the design of experiments. The second is that there is always some experimental error associated with the process of measurement; in the process of determining the value of some property of interest, the scientist must also provide a reasonable estimate of the likely error associated with the determination.

SAMPLES AND POPULATIONS

In the previous chapter we discussed ways of describing data derived from a sample of people or things, which are called "descriptive statistics." When you get those poor folks to imbibe gallons of clam juice, your hope as an experimenter is to infer some general rule about the effects of clam juice on patients with psoriasis that goes beyond the people who were actually involved in the study. In statistical jargon, you want to make inferences about the population based on the sample you have studied.

The statistical population has very little to do with our everyday notion of population, unless we're talking about census data or Gallup polls. The experimenter's population is the group of people about whom he wishes to make generalizations, patients with psoriasis, for example. In the best of all possible worlds, the experimenter should sample randomly from this population. In point of fact, this utopia can never be realized, if for no other reason than any experimenter who doesn't have a free pass on the airlines usually is constrained by geography to a particular area of the country, but it's often safe to assume that American psoriasis is the same as British psoriasis. Still, in the end it's up to the reader to judge the extent to which the results are generally applicable.

STANDARD ERRORS

The second major issue arising from this game of statistical inference is that every measurement has some associated error that takes two forms: systematic error and random error. An example will clarify this. Suppose, for some obscure reason, we wanted to determine the height of 14-year-old boys in the United States. That's our population, but no agency will fund us to measure all 14-year-old boys in the country, so we will settle for some samples of boys, for example, a random sample from 10 schools which were, in turn, randomly sampled throughout New York. Let's look at how our calculated mean height may differ from the true value, namely that obtained by measuring every boy in the United States and then averaging the results.

The idea of systematic error is fairly easy: if our ruler were an inch short or if the schools ended up with too many northern Europeans, then regardless of how large a sample or how many times we did the study, our results would always differ from the true value in a systematic way.

The notion of random error is a bit trickier, but fundamental to statistical inference. As an educated guess, the mean height of 14-year-olds is probably about 5'8", with a standard deviation of about 4 inches. This means that every time the experiment is performed the results will differ depending on the specific kids who are sampled. This variation in the calculated mean due to the fact that the individual measurements are scattered around the true mean value, is called "random error." Actually, statistics is lousy at dealing with systematic error, but awfully good at determining the effect of random error. To illustrate, if we just grabbed a few kids off the street, the chances are pretty good that some of them might be very short or very tall, and so our calculated mean may be quite far from the truth. Conversely, if we used thousands of kids, as long as they were sampled at random, their mean height value should fall pretty close to the true population mean. As it turns out, the mean values determined from repeated samples of a particular size are distributed about the true mean in a bell curve with a standard deviation equal to the original standard deviation divided by the square root of the sample size. This new S.D., describing the distribution of *mean* values, is called the standard error of the mean, or S.E.

$$\text{standard error} = \frac{\text{standard deviation}}{\sqrt{\text{sample size}}}$$

The exact way that the standard error is related to the standard deviation and sample size is shown in Figure 3.1.

Putting it another way, because every measurement is subject to some degree or error, every sample mean we calculate will be somewhat different. Most of the time they'll cluster fairly closely to the population mean, but every so often we'll end up with a screwball result that differs from the truth just by chance. So if we drew a sample, did something to it, and measured the effect we'd have a problem. If the mean differed from the population mean, is it because our intervention really had an effect, or is it because this is one of those rare times when we drew some oddballs? We can never be sure, but statistics tells a lot about how often we could expect the group to differ just *by chance alone*. More on this later....

INFERENCES ABOUT MEAN VALUES BASED ON A SINGLE SAMPLE

Let's try to clarify this basic idea in statistics by a specific illustration. Consider an experiment that may have a direct bearing on how well you under-

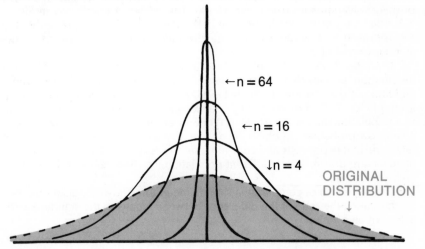

Figure 3.1 Original distribution and distribution of means related to sample size

stand what's to come. We have written the book on the assumption that the average reader has an IQ greater than 100. If we were wrong, then the readers may not be able to decipher these ramblings, and our royalties won't buy us a Big Mac®. So we'd like some reassurance that we've targeted the book about right. How will we test this hypothesis?

To begin with, we'll do as all good researchers are supposed to do by rephrasing it as a null hypothesis, that is to say, we'll start off by assuming that readers are no different in IQ than the population at large. We will then do our darndest to reject this hypothesis. So we phrase the null hypothesis:

$$H_o: \text{mean IQ of readers} = \text{mean IQ of general population}$$

We have deliberately chosen an experiment involving IQ tests since they are carefully standardized on very large samples to have a normal distribution with a mean of 100 and a standard deviation of 15. So when we state the null hypothesis, we are assuming, for the moment, that readers are a random sample of this population and have a true average IQ of 100. Sounds weird because that's just what we don't want to be the case, but bear with us.

Continuing along this line of reasoning, we then assume that if we were to sample 25 readers repeatedly, give them an IQ test, and calculate their mean score, these calculated means would be distributed equally around the population mean of 100. The question remains: what is the expected random variation of these mean values? Well, from the discussion in the previous section, the standard error of these means is just the standard deviation of the original distribution divided by the square root of sample size. In our case, this is $15/\sqrt{25} = 3.0$.

So, suppose we went ahead with the experiment involving 25 readers (we may have to give away a few complimentary copies to pull it off) and found their mean IQ to be 107.5. What we want to determine is the likelihood that we could obtain a sample mean IQ of 107.5 or greater from a random sample of the population with true mean of 100. This is shown graphically in Figure 3.2. What we are seeking is the area in the tail to the right of 107.5. The way we approach it is simply to calculate the ratio of (107.5–100) or 7.5 to the standard error of 3.0.

This ratio, $7.5/3.0 = 2.5$, tells us how far we are out on the standard normal distribution, and we then consult a table of values of the normal distribution, and find out that the area in the tail is 0.006. Thus, the likelihood of obtaining a sample IQ of 107.5 or greater by chance, under the null hypothesis that the two population means are equal, is 0.006 or about one in 160. Since there is a very low probability of obtaining a value this large or larger by chance, we reject the null hypothesis and conclude that the readers, with their average IQ of 107.5, are drawn from a different population, i.e., they really do have an IQ greater than 100.

This approach of comparing a sample mean to a known population mean by calculating the ratio of the difference between means to the standard error is known as a z test.

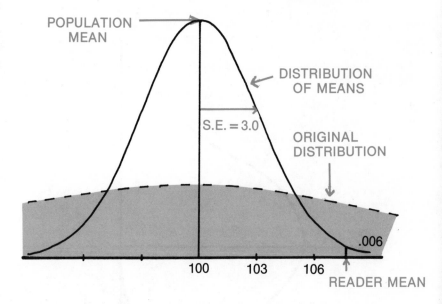

Figure 3.2   Distribution of mean IQ of sample size 25

Type I and II Errors, Alpha- and Beta-Levels, and Other Rules of Statistical Etiquette

The example we just worked through illustrates a couple of very basic rules of the game of statistical inference. The starting point is almost always to assume that there is no difference between the groups; they are all samples drawn at random from the same statistical population. The next step is to determine the likelihood that the differences you do observe could be due to chance variation alone. If this probability is sufficiently small, usually 1 in 20, then you "reject" the null hypothesis and conclude that there is some true difference between the groups. That is the meaning behind all those $p < 0.05$s and $p < 0.0001$s which appear in the literature. They are simply a statement of the probability that the observed difference could have arisen by chance. So you are concluding that the independent variable had some effect on the dependent variable and that therefore the samples came from different populations, the "alternative hypothesis" or H_1.

Going back to the "Reader IQ" experiment, we concluded that the population IQ of readers was greater than 100. Suppose, to carry on the demonstration, that it was actually 110 and not 107.5, the sample estimate. The distribution of sample means of size 25 drawn from the two populations, readers and general, could then be pictured as in Figure 3.3. The small area from the general population curve to the right of the sample mean is the probability that we could have observed a sample mean of 107.5 by chance under the null hypothesis. This is called the alpha (α)-level, the probability of incorrectly rejecting the null

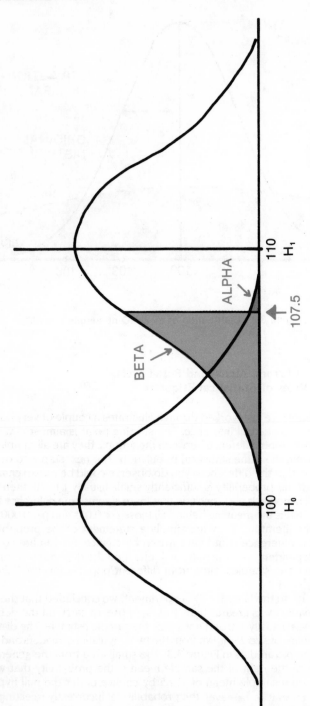

Figure 3.3 Alpha- and beta-errors

hypothesis, and the resulting error is called, for no apparent reason, a Type
I error. Of course, most statistical analysis uses an alpha-level of 0.05, which
means that there is one chance in 20 that they will conclude there is some difference when there isn't. This also means that of every 20 "significant" differences
reported in the literature, one is wrong. Wonder which one it is!

In analogous fashion, the area of the reader curve to the left of 107.5
represents the probability of obtaining a sample mean of 107.5 or less when
the true population mean is 110. This is called the beta (β)-level; the probability
of incorrectly accepting the null hypothesis when, in fact, the alternative hypothesis is true and this is of course a Type II error.

Conversely, the area to the right of 107.5 represents the probability that
a difference of 10 IQ points could have been detected in the experiment. This
probability, equal to $(1-\beta)$ is called the power. Among other things, power is directly related to sample size, since a larger sample size results in a smaller standard error, therefore less overlap of the two curves and more area to the right
of the sample mean. Figure 3.4 shows the relationship between power and sample size for various ratios of the difference to the standard deviation. Larger
sample sizes and higher z values (less overlap) result in greater power to detect
differences.

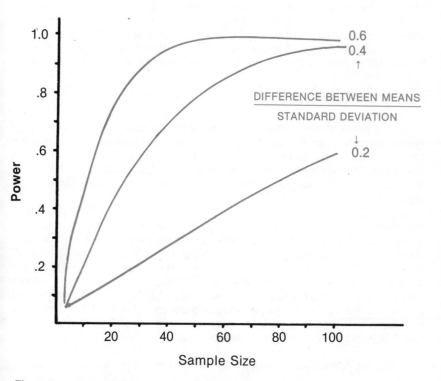

Figure 3.4 Relationship between power and difference between means standard
deviation and sample size

Up until now, we have only considered the possibility that readers were smarter than the general population. This conclusion would be accepted if the sample mean were sufficiently large that the probability in the right tail of the null hypothesis distribution was less than 5 percent. Since the hypothesis involves only one tail of the distribution, this is called a "one-tailed" test.

However the occasion may arise, for example in comparing two treatments, whereby we do not want to declare the direction of the difference ahead of time, but will be satisfied if a significant difference in either direction is obtained; so that if one treatment is better than or worse than the other by a sufficient amount, we will reject the null hypothesis. This amount must be determined by the probability in both tails of the distribution and so is called a "two-tailed" test.

What's the difference? In the two-tailed test, if we want to maintain an overall alpha-level of 0.05, we can allow only half this amount, or 0.025 in each tail. As a result, the difference between means must be larger in order to reject the null. For the z test, a difference of 1.64 standard deviations is significant at the 0.05 level for a one-tailed test, but a two-tailed test requires a difference of 1.96 standard deviations. This is illustrated in Figure 3.5

In real life, nearly all statistical analysis uses two-tailed tests. Even when comparing a drug to a placebo, people act as if they would be equally pleased to find that the drug is significantly better or worse than the placebo. The explanation for this bizarre behavior lies not in the realm of logic, but in political science. Apparently researchers, being an inherently conservative lot, don't want to go around rejecting null hypotheses with gay abandon. As a result, they go for two-tailed tests to stack the cards against them a little more.

CONFIDENCE INTERVALS

In the previous discussion, we put our data up against two hypotheses: (1) The mean population IQ of readers is 100, and (2) The mean IQ of readers is 110. Once the study is over, however, our best guess at the population IQ is not 100 or 110, but the value we determined from the study, 107.5. Nevertheless, there is some uncertainty in this estimate, which must be related to the standard error of the mean, 3.0.

This relationship is clarified in Figure 3.6. Imagine first that the true population mean were 1.96 standard errors below 107.5, or 101.6. In this instance, there is only a 2.5 percent probability that we could have obtained a sample IQ of 107.5 or more. Conversely, locating the upper boundary of the population IQ at 107.5 + 1.96 standard errors, or 113.4, there is a 2.5 percent probability that we could obtain a sample IQ as low as 107.5. Turning the whole argument around, we might say that having obtained a sample IQ of 107.5, there is a 95 percent probability that the true population IQ lies between 101.6 and 113.4. This range is called a "95 percent confidence interval," i.e., we are 95 percent confident that the population mean lies in this interval.

95 percent confidence interval = sample mean $\pm$ 1.96 $\times$ standard error

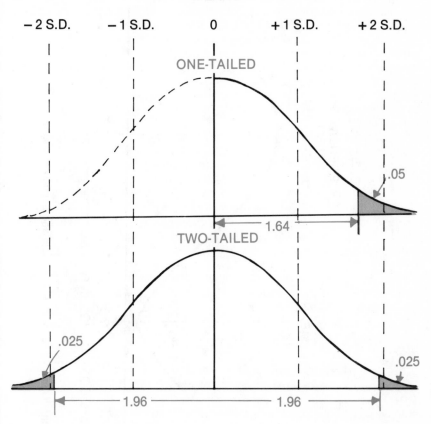

Figure 3.5 Comparison of One-tailed and Two-tailed Tests of Significance.

There is a natural link between the confidence interval and hypothesis testing. Looking at the figure, if the lower limit of the confidence interval was exactly 100, then the left-hand curve is identical to the null hypothesis distribution. So if the confidence interval includes the mean of the null hypothesis, then this is equivalent to not rejecting the null hypothesis.

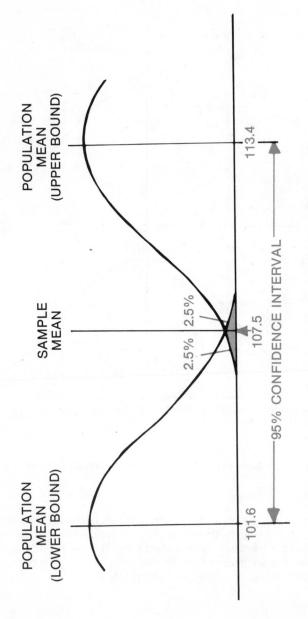

Figure 3.6 Confidence interval related to sample and population means.

STATISTICAL VS CLINICAL SIGNIFICANCE

In the preceding section we established the basic link between the magnitude of an observed difference and the calculated probability that such a difference could have arisen by chance alone. The game plan, then, is to determine this probability, and if it is sufficiently small, to conclude that the difference was unlikely to have occurred by chance alone. We then end up saying something like, "readers of the book are *significantly* smarter than the general population".

And that is the meaning behind statistical significance: that there was a sufficiently small probability of the observed difference arising by chance that we can conclude the independent variable had some effect. It's really too bad that in the history of statistics someone decided to call this phenomenon statistical significance as opposed to, say, "a statistically non-zero effect" or "a statistically present effect" because the term is, somehow, so significant. The basic notion has been perverted to the extent that $p < 0.05$ has become the holy grail of clinical and behavioral research, and $p < 0.0001$ is cause to close the lab down for the afternoon and declare a holiday.

Let's take a closer look at what determines that magical p level. Three variables enter into the determination of a z score (and as we shall see, nearly every other statistical test), (1) the observed difference between means, (2) the standard deviation of the distribution, and (3) the sample size. A change in any one of the three values can change the calculated statistical significance. As an example, we can examine the results of the Reader IQ experiment for sample sizes of 4 to 10,000. How would this variation in sample size affect the size of difference necessary to achieve $p < 0.05$ (i.e., statistical significance)? Table 3.1 displays the results.

TABLE 3.1   Relationship of Sample Size and Mean Values to Achieve Statistical Significance

Sample Size	Reader Mean	Population	p
4	110.0	100.0	0.05
25	104.0	100.0	0.05
64	102.5	100.0	0.05
100	102.0	100.0	0.05
400	101.0	100.0	0.05
2,500	100.4	100.0	0.05
10,000	100.2	100.0	0.05

So a difference of 10 IQ points with a sample size of 4 is just as significant, statistically, as a difference of 0.2 IQ points for a sample size of 10,000. We don't know about you but we would probably pay $100 for a correspondence course which raised IQ by 10 points (from 140 to 150, of course), but we wouldn't part with a dime for a course that was just as statistically significant, but only raised IQ by $\frac{2}{10}$ths of a point.

Sample size has a similar impact on the β-level. If the true IQ of readers was 110, a sample of 4 would have a β of 0.37, i.e., only a 63 percent chance of detecting it. The β-level for a sample of 100 is 0.05, and for a sample of 10,000 is less than 0.0001. So if the sample is too small, you risk the possibility of not detecting the presence of real effects.

The bottom line is this: the level of statistical significance, 0.05, 0.001, or whatever, simply indicates the likelihood that the study could have come to a false conclusion. By itself, it tells you *absolutely nothing* about the actual magnitude of the differences between groups.

Example 3.1

The Lipids Research Clinics (LRC) Trial screened 300,000 men to find 3,000 with cholesterol in the top 1 percent, no heart disease, and high compliance with the treatment regimen. They randomized the population to active drug and placebo regimens and, after 10 years, found 38 cardiac deaths in the controls and 30 in the drug group (p<0.05). A margarine company then proclaimed that everybody should switch from butter to margarine to prevent heart disease. Given your new knowledge, would you switch?

Answer:

This is a real perversion of the large sample. First, the effect of the drug is statistically significant, but clinically trivial in that the drug effect was real, but minimal for most patients. Second, the results may apply to folks similar to those studied, but don't apply to (a) women, (b) individuals with lower cholesterol levels, and (c) margarine users. This example, alas, actually occurred.

C.R.A.P. Detector #3.1

Beware the large sample. Effects can be statistically significant and clinically inconsequential.

C.R.A.P. Detector #3.2

Beware the sweeping generalization. Results of any study apply only to populations similar to the study sample.

Example 3.2

A rheumatologist studied the effect of copper brace-lets on 10 patients with arthritis. He measured 26 vari-ables and found a significant lowering of blood levels, but no effect on pain or function. He concluded that copper can affect blood levels of rheumatoid factor, but nothing else. Do you believe him?

Answer

Here's a small sample beauty. First, with 10 patients, he's unlikely to have enough power to show anything. So all he can safely say about the 25 other variables is that he was unable to demonstrate a difference and not that there wasn't one. Actually, you can never prove the null hypothesis. Second, with 26 tests, one may be significant by chance alone and so mean nothing.

C.R.A.P. Detector #3.3

Beware the small sample. It's hard to find significant differences, and no difference means nothing.

C.R.A.P. Detector #3.4

Multiple comparisons are a statistical no-no! There are special ways to handle these kind of data.

COMPARISON OF MEANS OF TWO SAMPLES: THE t TEST

> The t test is used for measured variables, in comparing two means. The *unpaired t test* compares the means of two independent samples. The *paired t test* compares two paired observations on the same individual or on matched individuals.

In our discussion of the z test we used a dependent variable, an I.Q. test, which has a known mean and standard deviation in order to compare our sample of interest, namely readers of this magnificant opus, to the general population. We did not have to scrape up a control group of non-readers for comparison because we know in advance the true mean and standard deviation of any control group we might draw from the general population.

This fortunate circumstance rarely occurs in the real world. As a result, many studies involve a comparison of two groups, treatment versus control, or treatment A versus treatment B. The statistical analysis of two samples is a bit more complicated than the previous comparison between a sample and a population. Previously, we used the population standard deviation to estimate the random error we could expect in our calculated sample mean. In a two sample comparison, this standard deviation is not known and must be estimated from the two samples.

Let's consider a typical randomized trial, say of an antihypertensive drug. We locate 50 patients suffering from hypertension, randomize them into two groups, institute a course of drug or placebo, and then measure the diastolic blood pressure. We can then go calculate a mean and standard deviation for each group. Suppose the results are as shown in Table 4.1.

Table 4.1   Typical Randomized Trial

	Treatment Group	Control Group
Sample size	25	25
Mean	98 mm Hg	102 mm Hg
Standard deviation	6 mm Hg	8 mm Hg

The statistical question is, "What is the probability that the difference of 4 mm Hg between treatment and control group could have arisen by chance?" If this probability is small enough, then we will assume that the difference is not due to chance, and there is a significant effect of the drug on blood pressure.

To approach this question, we start off with a null hypothesis that the population values of the two groups are not different. Then we try to show they are different. If we were to proceed as before, we would calculate the ratio of the difference between the two means, 4 mm Hg, to some estimate of the error of this difference. In the previous chapter, we determined the standard error, as the population standard deviation divided by the square root of sample size, but this time the population standard deviation is unknown. We do, however, have two estimates of this population value, the sample standard deviations calculated from the treatment and control groups. One approach to getting a best estimate of the population standard deviation would be simply to average the two values. For reasons known only to statisticians, a better approach is first add the squares of the standard deviations to give $6^2 + 8^2 = 36 + 64 = 100$. The next step is to divide this variance by the sample size and take the square root of the result to obtain the standard error:
error:

$$S.E. = \sqrt{(100/25)} = 2.0$$

As usual, then, to determine the significance of this difference, you take the ratio of the calculated difference to its standard error.

$$t = \frac{\text{difference between means}}{\text{standard error of difference}} = 4.0/2.0 = 2.0$$

The probability we are looking for is the area to the right of 8 mm Hg on a standard curve as shown in Figure 4.1.

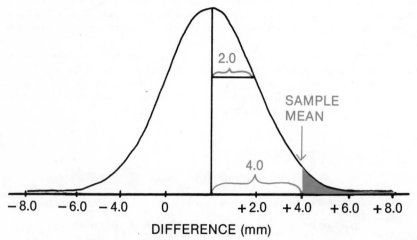

Figure 4.1 Graphical interpretation of the 't' test

This test statistic is called "Student's t." It was developed by the statistician William Gossett who was employed as a quality control supervisor at the Guinness Brewery in Dublin, and who wrote under the pseudonym of Student, presumably because no one who knew his occupation would take him seriously. It turns out that this curve is not quite a normal curve when you get to small samples, so you have to look it up in a different appendix, under the "t" distribution.

THE PAIRED T TEST

Before you knew anything about research design, you might have approached the hypertension trial somewhat differently. The most obvious way to do the experiment is simply to measure the diastolic pressure on a group of patients, give them the drug, and then measure the pressure again a month or two later. Suppose we measured five patients, whose raw data are represented in Table 4.2.

Table 4.2   Effect of Antihypertensive Agent on Diastolic Blood Pressure

Patient	Before	After	Difference
1	120.0	117.0	−3
2	100.0	96.0	−4
3	110.0	105.0	−5
4	90.0	84.0	−6
5	130.0	123.0	−7
Mean	110.0	105.0	−5.0
S.D.	15.8	15.7	1.58

Let's for a moment ignore the fact that these are before and after measurements, and assume they are data from two independent samples, with "before" representing the control group, and "after" the treatment group. If we were to proceed with a t test as described in the previous section, the difference between means is −5.0. The standard error of this difference is

$$S.E. = \sqrt{(15.8^2 + 15.7^2)/5.0} = 9.96$$

The t value then is −5.0/9.96 = −0.502, which is not significant.

However the samples are not independent but are paired observations of the same individuals before and after treatment. The right-hand column reveals quite a different picture. The average difference before and after is still −5.0. But the standard deviation of this difference, calculated as in any standard deviation, by squaring the differences between individual data and the mean average, dividing by the sample size minus one (more on this later), and then taking the square root, is only 1.58. The standard error of the difference is just $1.58/\sqrt{5.0} = 0.70$.

The test of significance used for this paired data is called a "paired t test," and is the ratio of the average difference (5.0) to the standard error of the difference (0.70).

$$t \text{ (paired)} = \frac{\text{mean difference}}{\text{standard error of differences}} = \frac{5.0}{0.70} = 7.14$$

This value is highly significant at the 0.00001 level.

How do we reconcile this major discrepancy between the two sets of results? If we back up from all the mathematical jimcrackery of the last page or so, and go back to the table of raw data, what the before-after observations succeed in doing is almost completely removing the effect of individual differences between subjects, resulting in an enormous increase in the precison of measurement.

It's easy to visualize any number of situations where individual patients could be assessed both before and after treatment. If we were looking at the effectiveness of a diet for treatment of obesity, it would be natural to weigh people before they started out on the diet and subtract this from their weight at the end. Similarly, if you want to try out an educational program to teach statistics to a heterogeneous group of health professionals, and assess its effectiveness with a multiple choice post-test, it would be a good idea to assess prior knowledge with a comparable pretest.

But it's worth a reminder that this experimental approach, although potentially more precise than a treatment-control group design, cannot ascribe the observed difference, statistically significant or not, solely to the experimental treatment. The weight watchers may have concurrently run out of food or developed an allergy to pizza, and the health professionals, in their enthusiasm, may have gone out and bought a copy of this book.

Example 4.1

Another true horror story. Several years ago, a popular treatment for angina was to ligate surgically the internal mammary artery. Patients rated the degree of pain before and after surgery. A t test showed significant reduction in pain as a result of surgery. The conclusion drawn was that the therapy was effective. Are you a believer?

Answer:

The small point is that the design demands a paired t test. When the test is not specified, it's usually unpaired, which is wrong. The big point, as shown later by randomized trials where the artery wasn't ligated in half the patients, was that the result was due to placebo effect. The moral is that you always need a control group to prove causation.

C.R.A.P. DETECTOR #4.1

To conclude that a difference between two groups, or a difference within a group, is due to some variable requires that the two samples differ only in the independent variable and none other.

COMPARISON AMONG MANY MEANS: ANALYSIS OF VARIANCE

> Analysis of variance (ANOVA) allows comparison among more than two sample means. *One-way ANOVA* deals with a single categorical independent variable (or factor). *Factorial ANOVA* can deal with multiple factors in many different configurations.

No doubt, on the occasions when you sat in front of your television set for an evening, it must have occurred to you to ask whether there really was any difference between products on the commercials. Is Cottonbelle™ really softer bathroom tissue, do floors shine better with new, clear, Smear™, does Driptame™ really stop postnasal drip? If you set out to do the experiment, one problem might be to pick two products to compare, since in the case of bathroom tissue, dirty floors, and runny noses there are many brand names to choose from. The real question is not so much, "Is Brand A better than Brand B?" but "Is there any measureable difference at all among the brands?" So instead of a single comparison between two groups, what we are after is some overall comparison among possibly many groups.

Let's be a bit more specific. Suppose as a family physician you are interested in determining whether there is a significant difference in pain-relieving characteristics among the many acetylsalicylic acid-based over-the-counter medications. A visit to the local drugstore convinces you to include six different medications in your study, five brand names and a generic drug. A first comparison you might wish to make would be between brand names and the generic drug, i.e., five possible comparisons. But you might also wish to compare Brand A to Brand B, A to C, A to D, and so forth. If you work it out, there are 15 possible comparisons. If there were 8 drugs there would be 28 comparisons; 10 drugs, 45 comparisons, and so on. The rub is that one out of 20 comparisons will be significant by chance alone, at the 0.05 level, so pretty soon you can no longer tell the real differences from the chance differences. The use of multiple t tests to do two-way comparisons is inappropriate, since the process leads to a loss of any interpretable level of significance. What we need is a statistical method that would permit us to make a statement about overall differences among drugs, following which we could seek out where the differences lie. Our null hypothesis (H_0) and alternative hypothesis (H_1) take the following form:

H_0 : All the means are equal.

H_1 : Not all the means are equal.

We would proceed to assemble some patients, randomly allocate them to the 6 treatment groups, administer the various ASA preparations, each delivered in a plain brown wrapper, and then ask the patients to rate pain relief on a subjective scale from 0 = no pain to 15 = excruciating. The results of the experiment are shown in Table 5.1.

Table 5.1   Pain Ratings for Patients in Six ASA Groups

Patient	Drug					
	A	B	C	D	E	F
1	5.0	6.0	7.0	10.0	5.0	9.0
2	6.0	8.0	8.0	11.0	8.0	8.0
3	7.0	7.0	9.0	13.0	6.0	7.0
4	8.0	9.0	11.0	12.0	4.0	5.0
5	9.0	10.0	10.0	9.0	7.0	6.0
Mean	7.0	8.0	9.0	11.0	6.0	7.0

Overall mean = 8.0

Five patients are assigned to each of the six groups. Each patient makes some pain relief rating (e.g., 5.0 is the rating of patient 1 in the drug A group). The mean relief in each group is obtained by simply averaging these ratings; 7.0 is the mean rating in group A. Finally, we can obtain an overall mean, 8.0 from averaging all 30 ratings.

Now, if we wanted to know whether drug A stood out from the crowd, the first step would be to find the difference between the mean pain score of drug A and the overall mean. Similarly, any difference between one drug and the rest can be detected by examining the difference between its group mean and the grand mean.

So to find the overall effect of the drugs, we take the differences between group means and the overall mean, square them (just as in the standard deviation) to get rid of the negative signs, and add them up. This sum looks like this:

$$(7-8)^2 + (8-8)^2 + (9-8)^2 + (11-8)^2 + (6-8)^2 + (7-8)^2 = 16.0$$

The sum is then multiplied by the number of subjects per group, 5, to obtain the sum of squares (between groups).

Sum of Squares (between) = sum of (group mean – grand mean)^2 × N

The next question is how to get an estimate of the variability within the groups. This is done by calculating the sum of the squared differences between individual values and the mean value within each group, since this captures individual variability between subjects. Because this is based on variation within groups it is called the sum of squares (within):

Sum of Squares (within) = sum of (individual value – group mean)^2

$$= (5\text{-}7)^2 + (6\text{-}7)^2 + (7\text{-}7)^2 + (8\text{-}7)^2 + (9\text{-}7)^2 +++ \dots (6\text{-}7)^2$$

There are 30 terms in this sum. The larger the sum of squares (between) relative to the sum of squares (within), the larger the difference between groups compared to the variation of individual values. However, the sums we calculated are dependent on the number of groups and the number of individuals in each group. To get around this one, the next step is to divide by the number of terms in the sum. Actually, at this point a little more sleight-of-hand emerges. Statisticians start out with the number of terms in the sum, then subtract the number of mean values which were calculated along the way. The result is called the degrees of freedom, for reasons which reside, believe it or not, in the theory of thermodynamics. Then dividing the sum of squares by the degrees of freedom results in a new quantity called the mean square. Finally, the ratio of the two mean squares is a measure of the relative variation between groups to variation within groups, and is called an F ratio.

F = Mean Square (between)/Mean Square (within)

This analysis is usually presented in an analysis of variance table, which looks something like this:

Table 5.2   Analysis of Variance

Source	Sum of Squares	Degrees of Freedom	Mean Square	F
Between groups	80.0	5	16.0	6.4
Within groups	60.0	24	2.5	
Total	140.0	29		

The first column lists the sums of squares over which we agonized. The second column includes the degrees of freedom, roughly equal to the number of terms in the sum of squares. The third column, mean square, derives from dividing the sum of squares by degrees of freedom. Finally, the F test is the ratio of the two mean squares, and can be looked up in yet another table at the back of the book. Because the method involves the analysis of only a single factor (e.g., drug brand), it is called One-Way ANalysis Of VAriance, or ANOVA.

These relationships may be presented graphically (Figure. 5.1). Individual data from each group are shown to be normally distributed around each group mean, and all groups are projected downward onto an overall distribution centered on the grand mean of 8.0. Now the mean square (between) is related to the average difference between individual group means and the grand mean, and the greater the differences between groups, the larger this quantity. The mean square (within) comes from the difference between individual data and their group mean, so estimates the variance of the individual distributions. Finally, the F ratio is the ratio of these two quantities, so the larger the difference between groups, in comparison to their individual variance, the larger the F ratio, and the more significant (statistically speaking) the result.

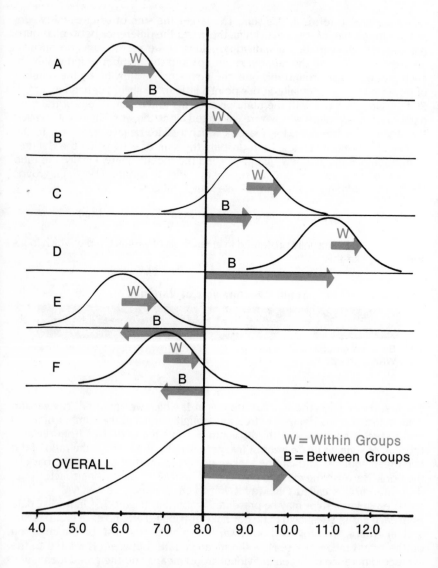

Figure 5.1 Graphical interpretation of one-way ANOVA

Let's go back to the initial question we posed. We wondered if there were any difference at all between various pain relievers. Having used ANOVA to satisfy ourselves that there is a significant difference somewhere in all that propaganda, the next likely question is "Where?" Note that if the ANOVA does not turn up any overall differences, the rule is: STOP—DO NOT PASS GO. DO NOT COLLECT $200. AND DO NOT DO ANY MORE NUMBER CRUNCHING. But supposing the F value was significant, there are a number of procedures, called "post-hoc comparisons" which can be used to find out where the significant differences lie. The use of a t test, even with a significant ANOVA, is still forbidden ground when there are many groups.

FACTORIAL ANALYSIS OF VARIANCE

If all ANOVA had to offer was a small edge over t tests in looking after significance levels, it wouldn't be worth all the effort involved in calculating it. But by an extension of the approach, called factorial analysis of variance, we can include any number of factors in a single experiment, and look at the independent effect of each factor without committing the cardinal sin of distorting the overall probability of a chance difference. As a bonus, we can also see whether, for example, some treatments work better on some types of subjects or have synergistic effects with other treatments, by examining interactions between factors.

To illustrate, let's examine that mainstay of midwinter television, the cough and cold remedy. Colds seem to come in two varieties, runny noses and hacking coughs. Some remedies like to take a broad spectrum approach: At last count, Driptame® was supposed to knock out 26 symptoms. Other brands try for specificity: Try-a-mine-ic® eats up about 6 feet of drugstore shelf space with all the permutations to make you dry up or drip more, cough less or cough loose. All in all, an ideal situation for factorial ANOVA. The original question remains: "Is there any difference overall among brands?" But some other testable questions come to mind. For example: "Do broad spectrum remedies work better or worse than specific ones?" "Which kind of cold is more uncomfortable?" "Do remedies work better or worse on runny noses or hacking coughs?" Believe it or not, it's possible to have a swing at all these questions at one time using factorial ANOVA.

Here's how. Start out with, say, 100 folks with runny noses and 100 others with bad coughs. Half of each group uses a broad-spectrum agent, and half a specific remedy. In turn, half of these groups get Brand A, and half get Brand B, or 25 in each subgroup. The experimental design would look like this:

Table 5.3 Experimental Design for Cold Remedy Study

	Broad Spectrum (BS)		Specific (SP)		
	A	B	C	D	Mean
Runny Noses (RN)	7.5	8.5	9.0	7.0	8.0
Hacking Coughs (HC)	4.5	5.5	5.0	11.0	6.5
Mean (Brands)	6.0	7.0	7.0	9.0	7.25
Mean (BS/SP)	6.5		8.0		

Now if we got everyone to score the degree of relief on a 15-point scale, the mean of RNs is shown as 8.0 on the right, and the mean of HCs is 6.5. Similarly, the mean for Brand A is at the bottom, 6.0, as are the other brand means. Means for BS and SP drugs are shown on the last line, and are just the averages of the two brands in each group. Finally, we have indicated all the individual subgroup means. Sums of squares for each factor can be developed just as before by taking differences between individual group means and the grand mean, squaring, and summing. This is then multiplied by a constant related to the number of levels of each factor in the design. For example, the sum of squares for Broad Spectrum versus Specific is:

$$\text{Sum of Squares (BS/SP)} = [(6.5-7.25)^2 + (8.0-7.25)^2]) \times 100 = 112.5$$

Mean squares can then be developed by dividing by the degrees of freedom, in this case 1, as we did before. But there is still more gold in them thar hills, called interaction terms. As discussed, one would hope that relievers that are specific for drippy noses work better in the RN group, and those specific to cough would be more helpful to HC members. That's an hypothesis about how the two factors go together or interact.

In Figure 5.2 we have displayed, on the left, the four cell means for the BS remedies. The center picture contains the cell means for the SP cures, and finally, the right graph looks at BS against SP by averaging across brands and plotting.

In the left picture, we see that overall the BS drugs are more effective for RNs than HCs (8.0 versus 5.0), and that Brand B has an edge of 1 unit on Brand A. But there is no evidence of interaction, since the lines are parallel. In the jargon, this overall difference is referred to as a main effect, in this case a main effect of Brand A and a main effect of RN–HC. By contrast in the middle picture, Brand C, which was specific for RNs, works much better for RNs, and Brand D for HCs. Overall, Brand D is only a bit better than C. So this picture shows a strong interaction, but little in the way of main effects. Finally, the right pic-

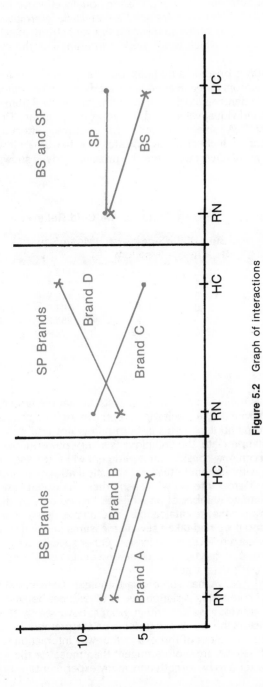

Figure 5.2 Graph of interactions

ture has a bit of both, since SPs and BSs are equally effective for RNs, but SPs work better for HCs. The important point is that useful information is often contained in the interaction terms, in this case the very strong effect of SPs if they are used as intended, which would be lost in examining the overall effect of each factor.

The calculations become a bit hairy, but the general principle remains the same. The numerators for each effect are based on squared differences among mean values. The denominators, or error terms, are derived from squared differences between individual values and the appropriate mean. The end result is an expanded ANOVA table with one line for each main effect and interaction and an F ratio for each effect which indicates whether or not it was significant. An example of an ANOVA table from the present study is shown in Table 5.4.

Table 5.4   ANOVA Table for the Cold Reliever Study

Source	Sum of Squares	Degrees of Freedom	Mean Square	F	p
RN/HC	112.5	1	112.5	4.10	<.05
BS/SP	112.5	1	112.5	4.10	<.05
BS/SP × RN/HC	112.5	1	112.5	4.10	<.05
Brand	125.0	2	62.5	2.27	NS
Brand × RN/HC	512.5	2	256.25	9.33	<.001
Error	5270	192	27.45		

The F ratio is really like all our other tests, in that the larger it is, the more statistically significant is the result. However,the associated probabilities are dependent on the number of terms in both numerator and denominator.

As you can appreciate, the technique is a very powerful one, albeit a little mysterious. You can now consider an experiment which tests several hypotheses simultaneously without committing any statistical atrocities, and you can look at how different factors interact with each other. The example we have chosen is one of semi-infinite number of possibilities, limited only by the imagination. Some of these variations are catalogued. For example, repeated measures ANOVA would be used if we had taken several measures on each subject by letting each subject try each reliever in succession. Other specific design terms include Latin square, split-plot, fractional factorial, and on and on, the specifics of which go far beyond our present needs.

But factorial ANOVA has some disadvantages. Conceptually it is still the familiar game of comparing variation due to differences between group means to variation of individual values within groups; however, by the time you get to four or five factors the results can become uninterpretable, because the differences are buried in a mass of three- and four-way interaction terms. Also, the assumptions of ANOVA are more stringent than those for the z test or for the t test, and these tend to be forgotten by many experimenters. In particular, the standard deviations within each cell of the design must be approximately equal. The design must be balanced, that is to say, there must be an equal number of subjects in each cell, or you cannot directly interpret the main effects and interactions.

Example 5.1

A study compared three different antacids for relief of gastric pain. The dependent variable was the pH of gastric contents after treatment. Twenty subjects, 10 male and 10 female, were in each group. A t test showed that C was better than A ($p < 0.05$), and better than B ($p < 0.001$), but there was no difference between A and B. Can you improve on the analysis?

Answer

First, the comparison of the three groups is just begging for a one-way ANOVA. However, if you used sex as a second factor, systematic differences between men and woman may emerge, as well as interactions. Finally, p values notwithstanding, the author has left us with no idea of the magnitude of the effect.

C.R.A.P. DETECTOR #5.1

Generally, there are more errors committed in not using ANOVA than in using it. Multiple comparisons demand ANOVA.

C.R.A.P. DETECTOR #5.2

Don't be misled by all the F ratios. Authors should still provide means and SDs so you can tell the magnitude of the effect.

C.R.A.P. DETECTOR #5.3

Generally, the use of multiple factors, which splits up the total variance among several independent variables, results in a smaller error term and a more powerful test.

RELATIONSHIP BETWEEN INTERVAL AND LINEAR REGRESSION, AND RATIO VARIABLES RELATED METHODS

> *Regression analysis* deals with the situation in which there is one measured dependent variable, and one or more measured independent variable(s). The *Pearson correlation*, and the *multiple correlation coefficient* describe the strength of the relationship between the variables.

Despite the fact that you have been introduced to some statistical sledge-hammers in the last few chapters, you might have noticed that conditions under which they could be applied were somewhat restrictive. One variable was always a nominal variable (reader/non-reader; clam juice/no clam juice) and the other variable was always interval or ratio. Although that describes the situation pretty well in many studies, there are two other combinations which frequently arise. The first is where both variables are nominal or ordinal (dead/alive; cured/not cured) in which case we must use non-parametric statistics. This situation will be dealt with in Section 3.

The second class of studies are those in which both independent and dependent variables are interval or ratio. This situation frequently arises when the researcher cannot institute an experiment in which some people get it and some don't. Instead, he must deal with natural variation in the real world, in which people may, of their own volition, acquire varying degrees of something, and then have more or less of the dependent variable.

For example, suppose you wanted to examine the relationship between obesity and blood sugar. In the best of all possible worlds, you would take a sample of newborn infants and randomize them to two groups. Group A members would be raised on pureed pizza, milkshakes, and potato chips for the next 40 years, and Group B constituents would have small quantities of rabbit food for the same period. But the ethics committee wouldn't like it, and the granting agency wouldn't fund it. So a more likely approach would be to venture timorously out into the real world, grab a bunch of complacent and compliant folks, measure their skinfold and blood sugar, and plot a graph depicting the relationship between them. If the relationship were really strong, these points would lie on a straight line. Unfortunately, these relationships don't occur very often in the real world since there are usually many variables, both known and unknown, which might affect blood sugar. So there is bound to be a great deal of scatter about the average line, and the first challenge may be determining where to draw the line.

If you recall your geometry, you might remember that a straight line equation is described as follows:

$$\text{blood sugar} = a + b \times \text{skinfold}$$

The y intercept of the line is "a," and "b" is the slope. The issue then is, "What is the best combination of "a" and "b" to yield the best fit?"

The way statisticians approach this is to define "best" in a particular way. They determine the vertical distances between the original data (•) in Figure 6.1 and the corresponding point on the line (0), square these distances, and sum over all the data points. They then select a value of "a" and "b" which results in the least value for this sum, what is called a least squares criterion. This sum of squares, which is an expression of the deviation of individual data from the best fitted line, is exactly analogous to the sum of squares (within) in ANOVA. A second sum of squares can then be calculated by taking the differences between the points on the line and the horizontal line through the two means, squaring, and adding. This one is analogous to the sum of squares (between) in ANOVA, and is called the sum of squares due to regression.

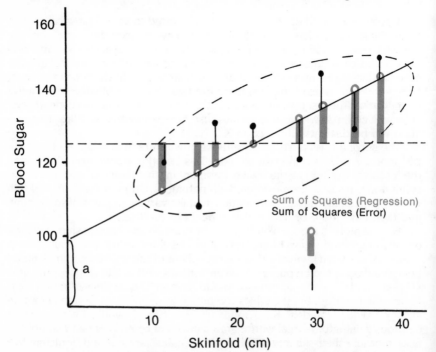

Figure 6.1 Relationship between blood and sugar skinfold

The strength of the relationship could then be expressed as the ratio of SS (regression) to [SS(regression) + SS(within)], expressing the proportion of variance accounted for by the independent variable. In fact, usually the square root is used, and is called a Pearson correlation coefficient.

$$\text{correlation} = \sqrt{\frac{\text{Sum of Squares (regression)}}{\text{Sum of Squares(regression)} + \text{Sum of Squares(error)}}}$$

The question of whether the relationship is statistically significant can be determined by looking up critical values of the correlation coefficient for a particular sample size. For example, for a sample size 20, a correlation of 0.44 or greater is significant at the 0.05 level. So if we had found a correlation of 0.5, we would conclude that there is less than 5 percent chance of a sample correlation coefficient occurring by chance, and that there is a significant relationship between the two variables.

We can interpret all this graphically by referring to Figure 6.1. In general, the individual data points constitute an ellipse around the fitted line. The correlation coefficient is related to the length of and width of the ellipse. A higher correlation is associated with a thinner ellipse and better agreement between actual and predicted values.

TWO OR MORE INDEPENDENT VARIABLES: MULTIPLE REGRESSION

In the previous example we dealt with the relationship between blood sugar and skinfold. This is the simplest form of regression analysis in that there is one independent variable, one dependent variable, and a presumed straight-line relationship between the two. A bit of reflection suggests that blood sugar is likely to be influenced by other variables, diet and heredity for example. If these could be used, it seems likely that our ability to predict blood sugar levels would improve. There is a fair amount of mileage to be gained by using several independent variables in predicting a dependent variable. The technique to do so is called multiple regression, and is an extension of the previous approach.

Suppose, for example, you are chairman of the admissions committee for the residency training program in pediatric gerontology at Mount Vesuvius Hospital. Every year you have interviewed all the applicants to the program, but you wonder if you might save some money and predict performance better using previous academic records. Performance in the program is based on a rating by supervisors. The academic record of applicants contains (1) grade point average in medical school (MDGPA), (2) National Board licence examination results (NBE) and (3) undergraduate grade point average (UGPA). The regression equation using these independent variables might look like this:

$$\text{performance} = a + (b \times \text{MDGPA}) + (c \times \text{NBE}) + (d \times \text{UGPA})$$

The statistical analysis, as before, is conducted by estimating values of the parameters $a \rightarrow d$ in such a way as to minimize the squared differences between the real data and the estimated points. Essentially, what the computer is doing is fitting a straight line in four-dimensional space (you will forgive us if we don't include a figure). And once again, the overall goodness of fit is determined by calculating a correlation coefficient from the ratio of the variance fitted by the line to the total variance. This correlation coefficient is called the multiple correlation (written R). The square of the multiple correlation can be interpreted directly as the proportion of the variance in the dependent variable, ratings, accounted for by the independent variables.

Of course, that isn't all the information obtained from the analysis. The computer also estimates the coefficients a to d, and does significance testing on each one. These coefficients indicate the degree of relationship between performance and each independent variable after the effects of all other variables have been accounted for.

Suppose, for example, that the resultant regression equation looked like this:

$$performance = 0.5 + (0.9 \times MDGPA) + (0.04 \times NBE) + (0.1 \times UGPA)$$

The estimated coefficients (0.9, 0.04, 0.1) are called unstandardized regression coefficients. Funny name since they look standard enough. It would appear that MDGPA predicts quite a bit, and NBE very little. But let's take a closer look. Suppose MDGPAs have a mean of 3.5 and standard deviation of 0.25. Then a change of one standard deviation in MDGPA results in a change of $0.9 \times 0.25 = 0.225$ in performance. By contrast, if NBE scores have a mean of 75 percent and standard deviation of 20 percent, a change of one SD yields a change in performance of $20 \times 0.04 = 0.8$ units in performance. So the size of the coefficient doesn't reveal directly how predictive the variable is. To make life easier, we often transform these to standardized regression coefficients or beta-weights, by converting each variable to have a mean of 0 and standard deviation of 1. The resulting weights can then be compared directly. In the present example, that would result in weights of 0.53 for NBE and 0.15 for MDGPA; thus, NBE is about three times as strong a predictor as MDGPA.

You might have your interest piqued by these results to explore the situation a bit further. For example, if you can do nearly as well without undergraduate GPA you might be prepared to forego this requirement. The question you now wish to ask is, "How much do I gain in prediction by adding in undergraduate GPA?".

One approach to this question would be to fit another regression line using only MDGPA and NBE, and determining the multiple correlation. The difference between the squared multiple correlations for the two equations, with UGPA in and out of the prediction, tells you how much additional variance you have accounted for by including the variable. This is the basic process in stepwise regression, a method where predictor variables are introduced one at a time into the regression equation, and the change in the multiple correlation determined. There are two ways of approaching stepwise regression: Either you can introduce the variables into the equation in some logical order specified by the experimenter, as in the current example, or you can let the computer decide the sequence.

The computer method is probably more popular. There are a number of esoteric criteria used to determine the order in which variables will be introduced. Basically, the computer will enter them in an order of decreasing ability to account for additional variance, a sort of statistical law of diminishing returns, so that at some point you can determine at what point little is to be gained by adding more predictor variables. The cutoff can be based on the statistical considerations that the contribution of an additional variable is not statistically significant. Alternatively, it can rest on more pragmatic grounds, namely that the additional explained variance isn't worth the effort.

Carrying the analysis of our example one step further, the data from the regression analysis might be presented in the style of Table 6.1.

Table 6.1   Results of Stepwise Regression Predicting Resident Performance

Step	Variable	Multiple R^2	Change in R^2	F Ratio	Significance
1	NBE	0.25		13.78	<0.0001
2	MDGPA	0.33	0.08	3.02	<0.05
3	UGPA	0.35	0.02	1.78	N.S.

The data show each step of the analysis on each successive line. The first step is just a simple regression, with the multiple R^2 equal to the square of the simple correlation $(0.50)^2 = 0.25$. The computer then calculated an F ratio, which proved to be statistically significant. At the second step, MDGPA was added, explaining an additional 8 percent of the variance and again this was statistically significant. Finally, introducing UGPA explained only 2 percent more of the variance, and was not significant.

One bit of subtlety. Sometimes a variable which has a high simple correlation with the dependent variable won't do anything in the multiple regression equation. Returning to our blood sugar example, an alternative measure of obesity might be kilograms above ideal weight, and it might correlate with blood sugar nearly as well as skinfold. But it's likely that the two are highly correlated, so if skinfold goes into the regression equation first, it is probable that kilograms won't explain much additional variance and may not be significant.

The message here is that a variable may not be a useful predictor of the dependent variable, for two reasons. One, it has a low correlation with the dependent variable. Two, it has a reasonable correlation with the dependent variable, but is highly correlated with another independent variable that has higher correlation with the dependent variable, and enters the equation first.

So that's what multiple regression looks like. Beware the study founded on a large data base but no prior hypotheses to test with an adequate experimental design. The investigators can hardly resist the temptation to bring up the statistical heavy artillery such as multiple regression to reach complex, glorious, and often unjustified conclusions about the relationships between variables.

Example 6.1

A large data base gathered over a 10-year period in a certain midwestern town (n = 12,498) was analyzed to determine predictors of high serum cholesterol. Twenty-eight different dietary factors were examined, and it was found that serum calcium levels correlated -0.07 ($p < 0.05$) with serum cholesterol levels. They concluded that low calcium causes high cholesterol. Will you drink more milk?

Answer

Not from these findings. A correlation of -0.07 is statistically significant because of the large sample, but accounts for only $0.07^2 = 0.49$ percent of the variance. Anyway, we would expect one of the 28 variables would be significant by chance alone. Finally, the association may be caused by something else.

C.R.A.P. DETECTOR #6.1

Beware the large sample revisited. With large samples, statistical significance loses all relationship to clinical significance.

C.R.A.P. DETECTOR #6.2

Watch out for fishing expeditions. The meaning of $p < 0.05$ applies equally well to correlation coefficients.

C.R.A.P. DETECTOR #6.3

Correlation does not imply causation. Height and weight are very highly correlated, but height doesn't *cause* weight. Researchers can get carried away when they see large correlations and start to interpret them as evidence of a causal relationship.

Example 6.2

A teacher of dyslexic children interviewed the parents of 12 of his students and found that birth order was significantly correlated with reading test scores ($R = 0.65$, $p < 0.05$). He concluded that lack of parent stimulation in infancy, which is more likely in large families, is a cause of reading problems. Agree?

Answer

There are a few difficulties here. With only 12 kids, one or two from very large families could bump up a correlation, significance notwithstanding. Also the fact that birth order was correlated with dyslexia does not imply a causative relationship.

C.R.A.P. DETECTOR #6.4

Beware the small sample revisited. It is easy to obtain correlations that are impressively large but cannot be replicated. A good rule of thumb is that the *sample size, or number of data points, should be at least five times the number of independent variables.*

C.R.A.P. DETECTOR #6.5

Regression equations may fit a set of data quite well. But extrapolating beyond the initial data set to values higher or lower is very tenuous.

C.R.A.P. DETECTOR #6.6

The multiple correlation is only an indicator of how well the initial data were fit by the regression model. If the model is used for different data, the fit won't be as good, simply because of statistical fluctuations in the initial data.

ANALYSIS OF 7 COVARIANCE

> Analysis of covariance (ANCOVA) combines both regression and ANOVA. There is one measured dependent variable. However, the independent variables can be both categorical factors and measured variables.

In the past few chapters we have developed a number of ways to analyze continuous data. *Factorial analysis of variance* deals nicely with the problem of nominal independent variables or factors, and *multiple regression* techniques deal with the case of several continuous predictor variables. All looks to be in fine shape.

Unfortunately, experiments in the real world are not quite so neatly categorized as these two techniques might suggest. A number of situations can arise where the independent variables may be a mixture of categorical and continuous variables, which cannot be dealt with adequately by either ANOVA or regression techniques. Here are some examples.

1. Examining the relative effectiveness of several drugs on subjective ratings of angina, adjusting for the degree of narrowing of coronary arteries, as measured by angiography.

2. Determining the relationship between dietary iron and hemoglobin levels, controlling for sex.

3. Predicting severity of arthritis measured by number of affected joints, from laboratory data including sedimentation rate (mm/hr) and rheumatoid factor (+/−).

In each of these situations, the dependent variable is continuous with interval data, but the independent variables are nominal with interval, continuous data. What is required is a statistical method that combines the best of both ANOVA and regression techniques. There are two approaches to dealing with this class of problems: Analysis of covariance (ANCOVA), and the general linear model or GLM. The latter is complex and rarely needed, so no more will be said of it here.

Suppose a psychiatrist decides to add one more study to the growing number that contrast one mode of psychotherapy with another. The two most popular methods to treat depression in middle age, the Tired Yuppie Syndrome (TYS), are Primal Scream (PS) and Hot Tub Hydrotherapy (HTH), and the outcome measure will be length of time in therapy. If he left it at this, things would be straightforward: Assemble a group of blue Yuppies, randomize to HTH or PS, count weeks in therapy, and do a t test on the means. But it is evident that his patients come in all shades of depression, from light blue to deep purple, and this is likely to affect outcome. So a better approach is to measure the degree of depression using a standard scale before starting therapy.

Now if HTH actually worked better than PS, resulting in fewer weeks of therapy, a plot of the dependent variable against the initial depression scores might look like the one depicted in Figure 7.1. The slope of the two lines indicates a linear relationship between degree of depression and time in therapy, and the vertical distance between the two lines is the relative effect of the two therapies. Finally, the error of the prediction is measured by the dispersion of individual points from the two lines.

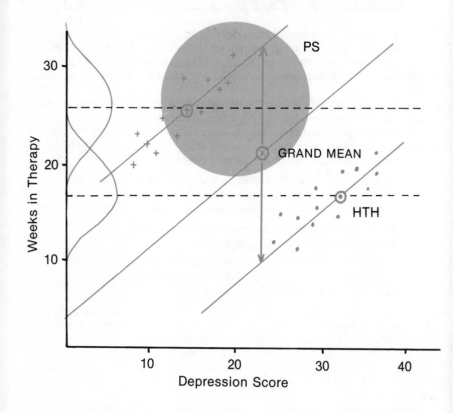

Figure 7.1 Relationship between initial depression score, treatment modality, and time in treatment

ANCOVA proceeds to fit the data with two lines, just as in regression analysis, estimating the slope of the lines and the difference between them. Statistical significance is tested by breaking up the total variation in the data into three components, as shown in the enlargement (Figure 7.2).

1. Sum of Squares due to regression (now called a covariate). This corresponds to the difference between the points on the fitted line and the corresponding horizontal line through the group mean. This is completely analogous to the regression case.

2. Sum of Squares due to treatments. This is based on the difference between the means in each group, and the grand mean, analogous to ANOVA.

3. Sum of Squares due to error. Just as with regression and ANOVA, this is merely the difference between the original data and the fitted points.

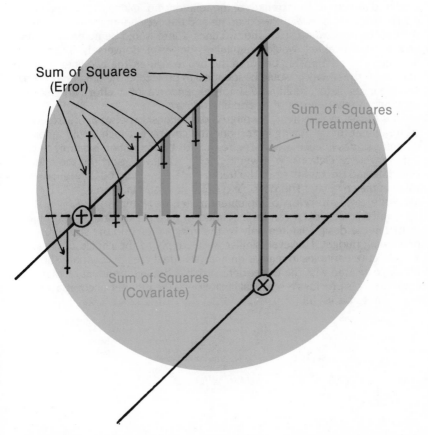

Figure 7.2   Enlarged view of ANCOVA showing sources of variance

Then by playing around with degrees of freedom and mean squares, F ratios are developed to determine whether each effect is significant. The results are displayed in a table similar to an ANOVA table, except that there is a separate line for the covariate.

Note what happens when all the data are projected onto the Y axis, as shown in Figure 7.1, which would be the case if the data were simply analyzed with ANOVA. First of all, because mean depression scores differed in the two groups, the projected means are much closer together, leading to an underestimate of the size of the difference between groups. Second, the dispersion of the data around the group means has increased by a factor of two or three. So a statistical test based simply on the differences between the group means could be biased and would be much less likely to detect a difference between groups than an ANCOVA. Turning it around, the potential advantages of ANCOVA are an increase in precision, hence an increase in the power to detect differences, and an ability to compensate for initial differences in the two groups.

However, this potential gain can only be realized if there is a relationship between the dependent measure and the covariate, and the gain in precision is related directly to the strength of the relationship. Taking the extreme cases, if the correlation between the covariate and the dependent measure were 1.0, then all the data would lie on the two lines. There would be no error variance, and the statistical test would be infinitely powerful. Conversely, if there were absolutely no relationship between the two measures, the two lines would be horizontal, the situation would be identical to projecting the data on the Y axis, and the investigator would have simply expended a lot of effort, and more importantly, a few degrees of freedom, to no avail.

It is a usual requirement that there is *no* relationship between the experimental treatment (the grouping factor) and the covariate, which would amount to different slopes in each group. The reason for this condition is simply because if there were a relationship, it would not be possible to sort out the effects of covariate and treatment, since the treatment effect would be different for each value of the covariate. This possible confounding is usually prevented by measuring the covariate prior to implementing the treatment.

The basic approach can be extended to multiple covariates and multiple factors in the design, limited only by the imagination and the size of the data processing budget. However, similar issues apply to the choice of covariates as predictive variables in regression analysis. Ideally, each covariate should be highly correlated with the dependent variable, but independent of each other covariate. This provides a practical limitation to the number of covariates which are likely to be useful.

Example 7.1

A psychologist got into a verbal exchange with a colleague over two modes of behavior therapy for patients with photonumerophobia.* He likes a gradual increase in exposure to the noxious stimulus, whereas his buddy throws his patients into the deep end, and then gives lots of support. To resolve the issue, they do a study in which the dependent variable is GSR (galvanic skin response), an index of anxiety, measured while subjects are delivering a research paper. After the lecture, subjects are then asked to recall how anxious they were before treatment, using a rating scale, to be used as a covariate. The covariate was significant (p < 0.05), but no treatment differences were found.

*Fear that their fear of numbers will come to light.

Question

Who wins the bet?

Answer

No one. Because the covariate was measured after treatment, people who responded well may rate their initial anxiety lower than those who didn't respond. Then if one method worked better, the final anxiety in this group would be lower, but so would the initial anxiety, leading to an underestimate of the treatment effect.

C.R.A.P. DETECTOR #7.1

Take a close look at when and how the covariate was measured and reassure yourself that it could not be confounded with the grouping variables.

C.R.A.P. DETECTOR #7.2

No amount of ANCOVA can safely adjust for initial differences between groups. Random allocation is better by far.

C.R.A.P. DETECTOR #7.3

Look closely at the size of the mean square of the covariate. If it's small, assume the researcher is just trying to dazzle you with statistical shotguns and doesn't know what he's doing.

TIME SERIES ANALYSIS

Time series analysis allows us to look at data where we make many repeated measurements on the same individual or organization over time. Because each value is correlated with the preceding and following data points to some degree, some special problems arise.

A topic closely associated with multiple regression is time series analysis (TSA). Both techniques attempt to fit a line (most often, a straight one) to a series of data points. However, while multiple regression examines how various independent variables operate together to produce an effect, TSA looks at changes in one variable over time. We do this in an informal and non-statistical way every day; in deciding whether or not to wear a coat today, we review the trend in the temperature over the past few days; or before investing the $20,000 we have just lying around gathering dust, we look at the performance of the stock market in general or of a specific company over the last few months. (We should note that some people rely on this "informal time series analysis" in situations where it shouldn't be used. After seeing four reds in a row at the roulette wheel, they bet more heavily on black, erroneously assuming that its probability of occurence is dependent on the previous spins. This is called the Gambler's Fallacy, and its perpetuation is fervently prayed for each night by casino owners.)

Although these examples may seem reasonable to a meteorologist or an economist, we rarely simply examine trends over time. More often, we are interested in a somewhat different question: Did things change after some *intervention*? Did the incidence of auto deaths fall after the speed limit was reduced? Was there a higher incidence of Guillain-Barré syndrome after the swine flu vaccination program was begun? Did the emptying of the psychiatric hospitals follow or precede the introduction of the phenothiazines? The technical term for this is an *interrupted* time series analysis, since we are examining the effects of an intervention which may interrupt the on-going pattern of events. The traditional way of representing this is

O O O O O X O O O O O

where the Os are observations of some variable over time, and the X represents the intervention. (We could of course use an I for the intervention, but this would be too logical.) This shows that we have two sets of observations, those made before the intervention and those made after it. Observations can be of a single person or event over time (such as the price of a certain stock for one year, or a child's behavior in a classroom during the semester), or each observation

71

can consist of the mean of different people or events (e.g., looking at how successive classes of applicants score on the MCAT).

These examples point to two major differences between multiple regression and TSA. First, in MRA, we are looking at the relationship between one dependent variable and one or more independent variables. In TSA, the interest is in changes in a single variable over time. One significant consequence is that in TSA the data are serially correlated. What this very impressive term means is that the value of the variable at Time 1 is related to and affects the value at Time 2, which in turn is related to and affects the Time 3 value. For example, today's temperature is dependent in part on yesterday's; it may differ by a few degrees one way or the other, but a large variation would be unexpected. Moreover, this implies that the temporal order of the variables is important; generally, the value for Time 5 must fall between those of Time 4 and Time 6, in order to make sense of the trend. Multiple regression is not designed to handle this serial dependency, and the order of the variables is quite arbitrary and does not affect the results. So regression should not be used to analyze time series data, although this has never stopped people from misapplying it in the past, and most likely will not stop them from doing so in the future.

When we are looking for the effects of some intervention, we can ask three questions: "Has the *level* of the variable changed?" "Has the *rate of change* of the variable changed?" "Have *both* the level and rate of change of the variable changed?"* "The easiest way to explain what these questions mean is through a few examples. To begin with, let's assume that we've just heard of a new golf ball that is guaranteed to shave five strokes from our game. How can we check this out? One way would be to play one game with our old ball, then one with the new ball, and compare scores. However, we know that the scores vary from day to day, depending in part on how we're feeling, but also because of our improvement (we hope) over time. So, any "positive" result with the second ball could be the result of a combination of natural fluctuations in our score, coupled with our expected improvement. What we need, therefore, is to play enough games with our first ball that we have a *stable* estimate of our score, then play enough rounds with the second ball to be confident we know our new average score. In Figure 8.1 we can see the variability in scores for the first six games played with the old ball and the latter six games played with the "new" ball. The arrow indicates when the intervention took place, and where we would expect to see an interruption in the time series. Our question would be: "Taking into account our slow improvement over time, and the variability in the two sets of scores, is the *level* of our scores lower, the same, or higher after the change?" Naturally, if there is a constant increase or decrease in the level of the scores, the average of the pre-intervention scores will always be different from the post-intervention average. So, when we talk about a "change in level," we compare the last pre-intervention score with the first one after the interruption. Before we tell you how we figure this out, we'll give a few more examples.

---

*There are also a number of other questions we can ask, such as: "Was the change immediate or was there a delay?" "Did it occur gradually or suddenly?" "Did it have a permanent effect or only a temporary one?" In fact, TSA can probably tell you more about the data than you really want to know.

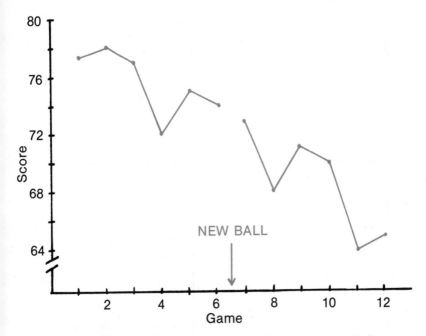

Figure 8.1   Golf scores before and after using a new ball

Despite what the drug manufacturers would like us to believe, there's some evidence that psychiatric hospitals began emptying out before the introduction of the major tranquilizers in 1955. If this is true, then we cannot simply look at the hospital census in 1954 and compare it with 1956, since the decrease may be due to reasons other than drugs. Our question has to be a bit more sophisticated: "Did the *rate* of emptying change because of the introduction of the psychotropic medication?" We can begin by plotting the total number of patients in psychiatric beds in the ten years prior to our time of interest, and for the following ten years, as we've done in Figure 8.2a. (Don't believe the actual numbers; they were made up for this graph.) Let's examine some possible outcomes. In Figure 8.2a, it appears as if the intervention has had no effect. The slope of the line hasn't changed, nor has the level of the line, following introduction of the new medication. In Figure 8.2b, there has been a sudden drop in the level, but the slope remains the same. This can occur if a large number of people were suddenly discharged at one time, but the steady outflow of patients is unchanged. For example, it's possible that, over the time span examined, the hospitals had begun keeping acute patients for shorter periods of time, so that their population began to drop. The new drug allowed the hospitals to discharge their previously untreated chronic cases within a short period of time, accounting for the sudden drop, but it did not hasten (or slow down) the steady discharge of other patients. Figure 8.2c shows the situation where the rate of discharge was speeded up by the new drug, but without a mass discharge of patients at one time. Lastly, Figure 8.2d shows both effects happening at once, namely a sudden discharge of patients followed by an increased discharge rate

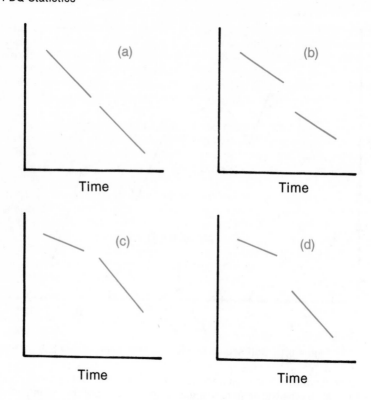

Figure 8.2 Different possible results from an intervention

for the remaining patients. These are not the only possible patterns; let your imagination run wild and see how many others you can dream up. Try adding a delayed effect, a temporary effect, a gradual effect, and so on.

Let's turn our attention from *what* TSA does to *how* it achieves such miracles. One factor which makes our job of interpreting the graph more difficult is that the value of the variable may change over time, even without any intervention. If the change is always in one direction, it is called a trend. A gradual change one way followed by a gradual change the other way is referred to as drift. If we have relatively few data points, it may be difficult to differentiate between the two. The primary cause of trend or drift is the dependency of a value at one point upon previous values. As we mentioned before, this is called serial dependency, and we find out if it exists by calculating the autocorrelation coefficient. When we compute a normal run-of-the-mill correlation, we have two sets of scores, X and Y, and the result can tell us how well we can predict one from the other. The "pairs" of scores are formed somewhat differently in autocorrelations; the value at Time 1 is paired with the value at Time 2, Time 2 is paired with Time 3, and so on. In an analogous way with a Pearsonian correlation, this tells us to what degree scores at time t are predictive of scores at time $t+1$, and is referred to as a lag 1 autocorrelation. However, the effect at time t may be powerful enough to affect scores down the line. We can explore this by lagging the scores by two units (e.g., Time 1 with Time 3, Time 2 with Time 4), three units (Time 1 with 4, 2 with 5), and so forth. If the lag 1 autocorrelation is significant (i.e., if the data *are* serially dependent), then the autocorrelations most often become smaller as the lags get larger. This makes sense on an intuitive level, since the effect of one event on subsequent ones usually dissipates over time.

A significant autocorrelation can be due to one of two causes: the scores themselves may be serially correlated, or sudden "shocks" to the system may have effects which last over time. The first situation is called the autoregression model, while the second is referred to as the moving averages model. Thus, this is known as the autoregressive integrated moving averages (ARIMA) technique. Moving averages is another trick of the statisticians to smooth out a messy line, one with fluctuations from one observation to the next. We can take the average of scores 1 and 2, then the average of 2 and 3, then of 3 and 4, and so on. If the curve hasn't been smoothed enough, we increase the *order* of smoothing, by averaging scores 1, 2, and 3; then scores 2, 3, and 4; 4, 5, and 6; until the end of the series. Since the extreme score is "diluted" by averaging it with more "normal" ones, its effect is thereby lessened. Theoretically we can continue this until we have only one number, the mean of all of the scores.

Our next step is to try to remove the effect of the trend or drift, in order to see if there is any change in the level. This is done by differencing the time series, which means that the observation at Time 1 is subtracted from the one at Time 2, Time 2 is subtracted from Time 3, and so forth. Let's see how this works. Assume we have the sequence of numbers

1   3   5   7   9   11   13

If we were to draw these on a graph, a definite trend is apparent since the points would increase in value with every observation period. Now, let's take the differences between adjacent pairs of numbers. What we get is

2   2   2   2   2   2

where it's obvious that there is no trend: The line is flat over all the observations. Note two things: First, there is one less differenced number than original observations. Second, and more important, life is never this beautiful or clean-cut.

The success of differencing is checked by recalculating the autocorrelation. If it worked, then the autocorrelation should quickly (i.e., after a few lags) drop to zero, and the series is said to be stationary. If there is still a trend, we repeat the process by subtracting the first differenced value from the second, the second from the third, and so on. Although in theory we can repeat this process of autocorrelating and differencing many times (or at least until we run out of numbers, since we lose one observation each time we difference), in practice we need only do it once or twice.

Up to this point, what TSA has done is to try to determine what factors can account for the data, by going through a sequence of steps:

1. Compute the lagged autocorrelations to determine if the sequence is *stationary* or *non-stationary*.

2. If it is non-stationary, *difference* the scores until it becomes stationary.

3. Recompute the autocorrelations to see if the trend or drift is due to an *autoregressive* or a *moving averages* process.

These steps are referred to collectively as model identification. The next stages involve actually trying out this model with the data to see how well they fit. This involves *estimating* various parameters in the model and then *diagnosing* where any discrepancies are. This again is an iterative process, since any discrepancies suggest we have to identify a new model, estimate new parameters, and again diagnose the results.

Once all this is done we can move on to the last step, which is to see if the intervention had any effect. One way of doing this is simply to analyze the pre- and post-intervention data separately, and then to compare the two models. The parameters will tell us if there has been a change in the trend, in the level, or in both. We are fortunate in that computer programs exist to do the work for us, although this is a mixed blessing since it has allowed people to analyze inappropriate data and report results that best belong in the garbage pail.

Example 8.1

It has been suggested that even brief psychotherapy can reduce medical utilization. To test this out, a researcher looks at the total dollar expenditure on health care in a group of patients for each of the 12-month periods prior to and after therapy.

Question 1

Can these data be analyzed with a time series analysis?

Answer

The *type* of data are appropriate for TSA, but there are too few data points. In order to get a stable estimate of the parameters, she should have had at least 30 (yes, 30) observations in each set. Lately there seems to be a contest to see who can analyze the sequence with the fewest number of points. This is an extremely unfortunate trend (pardon the pun), since this technique clearly is inappropriate with fewer than 30 observations, especially if there are wide fluctuations from one point to another.

C.R.A.P. DETECTOR #8.1

In TSA, look for at least 30 pre- and post-intervention measurements.

Question 2

Her conclusions read simply that, "A time series analysis showed significant changes after a course of therapy." What's missing?

Answer

What model did she use? Autoregressive? Moving averages? Another? With so many options, the researcher must tell us what assumptions were made before we may accept the conclusions drawn by statistical methods.

C.R.A.P. DETECTOR #8.2

If the author does not state if the data were differenced, or whether an autoregressive or a moving averages model was used, don't bother reading further. If the model was specified, the author must give the reasons for using one model rather than another.

NON-PARAMETRIC STATISTICS

NON-PARAMETRIC TESTS OF SIGNIFICANCE

9

> A variety of statistical tests have been devised to ex-
> amine the association between a single categorical
> independent variable and nominal or ordinal depen-
> dent variables. These include the *chi-square, binomi-*
> *al test*, and *Fisher exact test* for nominal data and
> independent samples; the *McNemar chi-square* for
> related samples; the *Mann-Whitney U*, the *Median*
> test, the *Kruskal-Wallis* and the *Kolmogorov-Smirnov*
> test for ordinal data and independent samples, and
> the *Sign test* and *Wilcoxon test* for ordinal data and
> matched samples.

Although quantitative measurement is essential to the biological disciplines
that are the basis of the health sciences, clinical research is often more con-
cerned with the practical issues of preventing disease, treating illness, and
prolonging life. The object of measurement, in turn, is the determining the
presence or absence of risk factors, assessing the presence or absence of particular diseases, and estimating survival (the presence or absence of death).
These measures are all nominal categories, and the numbers are body counts;
(e.g., the number of people with angina, treated with a beta-blocker, who sur-
vived 1 year). These kinds of data require different kinds of statistical methods,
called non-parametric statistics for analysis. By far the most common non-
parametric test is the chi-square test.

TESTS FOR NOMINAL DATA

For example, there has been a great deal of discussion recently about the
possible adverse health effects of video display terminals (VDTs). Since this book
is written on a VDT, the question is of more than passing interest. One factor
that clouds the issue is that the people who are most exposed are also in pressure cooker jobs, so stress may be the real problem. To put it
to the test, how about examining a different form of VDT, the kind which popu-
lates video arcades and is strictly for recreation. Because the adverse health
effects seem to be rare, we might go for a case-control design: First locate a
group of young mothers who experienced complications of pregnancy, then compare them to a group with normal deliveries on the basis of time spent in video
arcades during pregnancy. The data might look like those arrayed in Table 9.1.

Table 9.1   Association of Pregnancy Complications in Young Women and the VDT Exposure in Video Arcades

Exposure	Complicated Pregnancy	Normal Pregnancy	Total
Yes	60	50	110
No	40	150	190
	100	200	300

If exposure had no effect, we should expect that the proportion of individuals in both groups who had been in arcades would be the same. The best guess of this proportion is based on the sum of both groups, 110/300 or 37 percent. So the expected number exposed in the cases is just 0.37 × 100 or 37, and the control group is 0.37 × 200 = 74. Similarly, the expected frequencies in the bottom two cells are 63 and 126.

CHI SQUARE

One way to test the statistical significance of the association is to determine the difference between the observed and expected frequencies, and proceed as we have done many times before to create a variance term by squaring them and adding them up:

$$(60-37)^2+(50-74)^2+(40-63)^2+(150-126)^2$$

The usual approach now would be to go looking for some way to estimate the standard error of the differences to use as a denominator. In contrast to our previous examples, we don't have any individual values in each cell to estimate the standard deviation, just a single number. But fortunately, Mother Nature comes to the rescue. It turns out that as long as the expected frequencies are fairly large, they are normally distributed, with a variance equal to the frequency itself. For an expected frequency of 16, the variance is 16, and the standard deviation is 4. Because the variance is simply the expected frequency in each cell, the approach is to divide each term separately by its expected frequency. The test looks like this:

$$\frac{(60-37)^2}{37}+\frac{(40-74)^2}{74}+\frac{(40-63)^2}{63}+\frac{(160-126)^2}{126}=47.49$$

That ratio is called chi-square or X^2, the most commonly used non-parametric test by a long shot. The larger its value, the more the numbers in the table differ from those we would expect if there were no association. So chi-square is a test of the association between two variables. It can easily be extended to more than two levels for each variable. For example we could have defined time in the video arcades as high, low, or none, resulting in a 2×3 table.

The bad news is that it has a few limitations. The first is that it assumes no ordering among the categories, but treats the categorical variable as nominal. That's okay if it is a nominal variable, but if the categories are ordered, there's information that isn't being used by the test. A second problem is that when the expected frequency in any cell is small—less than 5 or so—the test is inaccurate.

The two alternatives that can be used with analyses with small expected frequencies are both based on calculating the exact probability that the particular frequencies which were observed could occur by chance. Both tests yield exact answers, even when frequencies in some cells are zero, but they can only be applied under very restricted circumstances.

THE BINOMIAL TEST

The binomial test is a one-sample test, like the z test in parametric statistics. In addition, it is restricted to only two cells.

Suppose we had six patients with a very rare disease, Tanganyikan Restaurant syndrome. Detailed statistics collected by the previous British Raj indicate a survival rate of 50 percent. After a course of therapy consisting of pureed granola and wild bee honey, 5 patients remain alive. Is this a statistically significant improvement in survival?

If the expected survival rate is 50 percent, then the likelihood that any one patient would survive is 0.5; so the probability that all six patients would survive is $0.5^6 = 1/64$. With a little more probability logic, we can see that there are six ways 5 out of 6 would survive: patient 1 dies and the rest live, patient 2 dies and the rest live, and so on. The probability of any one outcome is still 0.5^6, so the probability of 5 survivors is $6 \times 0.5^6 = 6/64$. Since we are trying to reject the null hypothesis, we want to determine the likelihood that 5 survivors, or any more extreme numbers, could arise by chance if the expected number of survivors were 50 percent or 3. Thus, the overall probability of 5 or more survivors, under the null hypothesis, is $6/64 + 1/64 = 7/64$, which is not significant. So we would conclude in this example that there has not been a significant decrease in fatality rate.

The approach can be extended to other expected probabilities by some fancier formulas, but the approach of adding up the exact probability of the observed, and all more extreme possibilities, remains the same.

That's the binomial test. Again, a reminder that the binomial test is a useful replacement for X^2 when the expected frequencies are less than 5, but it only works for a single sample with two cells.

FISHER EXACT TEST

The equivalent exact test to the binomial test for the case of two independent samples is the Fisher exact test. Like the binomial test, it is a useful replacement for X^2 when the expected frequencies are small. Also like the binomial test, the Fisher exact test permits only two responses.

A common situation where Fisher's test must be used is in the analysis of trials where the outcome of interest, such as death, occurs fairly infrequently.

Since there is some suggestive evidence that alcohol may reduce the rate of heart disease, how about a trial where half the folks get vodka with their orange juice and half don't. Five years later we look at cardiac deaths, and see the following results:

**Table 9.2A Comparison of Cardiac Death Rates
(Vodka Drinkers and Non-drinkers)**

	Vodka Drinkers	Control	Total
Alive	197	192	389
Dead	3	8	11
Total	200	200	400

The null hypothesis is that there is no difference in the proportion of deaths in the two groups. A chi-square test cannot be used because the expected frequencies in the two bottom cells are too small (i.e., 5.5) so it's necessary to use an exact test. A complicated formula exists to calculate the exact probability from probability theory. But to test the null hypothesis, you also have to determine the probability of all the more extreme values. To get at the more extreme values, you keep the marginal values fixed (keep the totals of each row and column, i.e., 200, 200, 389, and 11, the same) and reduce the value in the smallest cell by one until it is zero. In our example, the more extremes, keeping the same marginals are:

Table 9.2B Effect of Vodka Consumption on Cardiac Death Frequency

	Vodka Drinkers	Controls	Vodka Drinkers	Controls	Vodka Drinkers	Controls
Alive	198	191	199	190	200	189
Dead	2	9	1	10	0	11

It's simply a case of sticking these three combinations into the formula, which determines the probability of occurrence of each combination by chance, adding up the probabilities, and concluding whether the total probability is sufficiently small to reject the null hypothesis.

THE McNEMAR TEST

As the chi-square and the Fisher test are to the unpaired t test, so the McNemar test is to the paired t test. It is used for two related measures on the same sample, or other situations where each individual measurement in one sample can be paired with a particular measurement in the other. The ordinary chi-square test assumes independence of sampling in the two groups and therefore cannot be used at all when the two samples are matched. The McNemar test is a modification of chi-square which takes into account the matching of the samples.

As we write this section, we are immersed in yet another election campaign. As usual, both major political parties are assaulting the voter's senses with television commercials showing the party leader, every hair in place, pearly white teeth gleaming, surrounded by equally handsome happy people and delivering with gusto the message that either (a) the economy has never been better (party in power), or (b) the economy has never been worse (opposition party). One wonders whether the ad men ever bothered trying to find out if these inane bits of fluff could change anyone's mind. It would be easy to do. You could grab 100 folks off the street, find out their political allegiance (if any), inflict the commercial on them, and see if any change has resulted. The data might look like:

| | | AFTER | |
		Donkey	Elephant
BEFORE	Donkey	35[a]	15[b]
	Elephant	10[c]	40[d]

Figure 9.1   Effect of television commercial on party allegiance

Note that the only people on whom the commercial had any effect are those in cells (b) and (c). As a result of the commercial, 15 people changed from Donkeys to Elephants, and 10 the other way. It is these cells on which we will focus.

Under the null hypothesis of no effect, we would expect that as many people would change in one direction as the other. That is to say, the expected value of each cell is

$$\frac{(b+c)}{2} = \frac{25}{2} = 12.5$$

From here on in, it's easy. We simply use the observed values in the changed cells and these expected values, in a chi-square calculation.

$$\text{Chi-square} = \frac{(15-12.5)^2}{12.5} + \frac{(10-12.5)^2}{12.5} = 1.0$$

This is distributed, more or less, as a chi-square distribution, with one degree of freedom. It turns out that a better approximation to chi-square, for mysterious reasons, is determined by subtracting one from the numerator, and after some algebra we get:

$$\text{Chi-square} = \frac{(b-c-1)^2}{(b+c)} = \frac{(15-10-1)^2}{25} = 0.64$$

Compare the X^2 value with table to determine significance and that's the McNemar Test. Since the value was not significant, we would conclude that neither was the commercial.

NON-PARAMETRIC TESTS ON ORDINAL VARIABLES

In previous chapters we have made the point that the use of non-parametric tests on data which are interval or ratio is akin to throwing away information. Similarly, applying a test such as chi-square to data which can be ordered can also result in a loss of information.

A wide variety of non-parametric tests can be applied to this situation. For some bizarre reason, nearly all of these tests were developed by two-man teams, unlike the one-man shows of Fisher, Pearson, and Student. In this section we're going to have a look at a series of partnership efforts: Mann and Whitney, Kolmogorov and Smirnov, and Kruskal and Wallis.

As an example, let's use the old favorite of pain researchers, the visual analog scale (VAS). The scale is a 10 cm line with labels such as "Depressed and Near Death" at one end and "Happy and Healthy" at the other. The patient simply puts an "X" on the line indicating how he or she feels. As usual, the title does much to make the method look more sophisticated than it is. Even though you can measure a score to a millimeter or so, there really is no assurance that the psychological distance between 9 cm and Healthy (10 cm) is the same as that between Death (0 cm) and 1 cm, so there is some reason to treat these data as ordinal. (The same comments apply to nearly any rating scale if you want to be hard-nosed about it.)

Judging from the commercials, hemorrhoids produce the kind of pain amenable to do-it-yourself solutions. How about a trial of Preparation Help and a placebo (Preparation P). We mail one tube each to 20 of our suffering friends, so that 10 receive H and 10 P, with a VAS to fill out. The data might look like this:

Table 9.3   Pain Scores for Hemorrhoid Preparations

	H			P	
Subject	Score	Rank	Subject	Score	Rank
1	9.8	1	11	8.6	5
2	9.6	2	12	8.2	7
3	8.9	3	13	7.7	9
4	8.8	4	14	7.5	10
5	8.4	6	15	6.9	12
6	7.9	8	16	6.7	13
7	7.2	11	17	4.9	17
8	5.8	14	18	4.5	18
9	5.5	15	19	3.5	19
10	5.1	16	20	1.5	20

If these were interval data, then we could simply calculate means and standard deviations, plug them into a formula, and calculate results using the usual t test. But if we aren't prepared to assume that the data are interval, then some other approaches are necessary. Most are based on rank-ordering of the combined data, one way or another, and then performing the gimcrackery on the ranks. We have taken the liberty of adding combined ranks to the table, for further use.

THE MANN-WHITNEY "U" TEST

The U test looks at the relative ranks of subjects in the two groups. Collapsing the ranks together, and labelling the origin of each subject by H or P, they look like this:

Rank	1	2	3	4	5	6	7	8	9	10	11	12	13	14	15	16	17	18	19	20
Group	H	H	H	H	P	H	P	H	P	P	H	P	P	H	H	H	P	P	P	P

Now if H were truly better, then most people would give it a higher rank, all the Hs would be on the left, and all the Ps on the right.

We develop a total score, called U naturally, from the total number of times an H precedes each P. If all Hs were ranked more highly, then each P would be preceded by 10 Hs. If things were totally interspersed, then on average each P would have 5 Hs above it and 5 below. In this case, the first P has 4 Hs ahead, adding 4 to the sum. The next P has 5 ahead, and the the next has 6. Working this through the lot, the sum comes out as follows:

$$4 + 5 + 6 + 6 + 7 + 7 + 10 + 10 + 10 + 10 = 75$$

We then rush to the appropriate table, which probably kept Mr. Mann and Mr. Whitney busy at their calculators for years, and look up our figure of 75 to see whether it is big enough to be significant. It turns out that it isn't. There are some additional wrinkles which are introduced if the sample size is very large, and if there are tied ranks (i.e., two scores exactly the same), but what we have described is the basic U test.

THE MEDIAN TEST

If we went back to our original data, we could determine that the median score of the entire sample of scores was 7.5. It is fairly straightforward to determine how many in each group are above and below the median. The data end up in a 2 × 2 table:

	H	P	Total
Above Median	7	3	10
Below Median	3	7	10
Total	10	10	

Figure 9.2   2 × 2 Table comparing treatment versus control data

This can be analyzed in the same manner as any 2 × 2 table, using chi-square or the Fisher exact test. In this case, the Fisher exact test is appropriate since the expected frequencies in all cells are exactly five. As it turns out, the test is not significant.

It's no surprise that the median test isn't associated with any two-man team. It is a commonsense thing to do if you want to analyze ordinal data with a chi-square statistic, and the only mystery is how the approach managed to achieve sufficient eminence to find a place all by itself in statistics books.

THE KRUSKAL-WALLIS ONE-WAY ANOVA BY RANKS

As we indicated earlier, one way of straightening out the curves in ordinal data is to convert the original data into ranks. The data in each group would then look like the two Rank columns. If there are differences between H and P, the average rank in the two groups would differ, and we could proceed to analyze the ranks by ANOVA. It turns out that the use of ranks results in some simplifications in the formulas, so that after the dust settles, the equivalent of an F test becomes:

$$H = \frac{12}{N(N+1)} \times \frac{\text{sum of (total rank in groups)}^2}{\text{Number in group}} - 3(N + 1)$$

where N is the total number of observations.

In this example, the total rank of the Hs is 80 and of the Ps is 130. The formula becomes:

$$H = \frac{12}{20\,(21)} \times \frac{(80^2 + 130^2)}{10} - 3 \times 21 = 3.57$$

This is distributed as a chi-square with degrees of freedom equal to the number of groups less one. In our example, the probability is between 0.10 and 0.05, nearly significant.

Note also that the test, like the median test is not restricted to two groups, but can be applied to any number of groups. By the way, all three tests are subject to the same limitations of small numbers as the chi-square test. In the median test, if the expected value in any cell is less than 5 (i.e., any group less than 10) then the investigator should analyze the frequencies with the Fisher exact test. In the Kruskal-Wallis test, if any of the sample sizes in a group is less than 5, then you have to go to a special table of exact probabilities.

THE KOLMOGOROV-SMIRNOV TEST

Let's take one last run at this data set. The Kolmogorov-Smirnov test capitalizes on a cumulative frequency distribution, a term which may be unfamiliar but which can be easily understood through our example. If we were to classify the raw scores of the two samples in groups such as 5.6–6.0, 6.1–6.5, ... 9.6–10.0, then it is straightforward to count the number of subjects in each group who fall in each category (i.e., to develop a frequency distribution).

These frequencies can then converted into a probability distribution by dividing by the sample size in each group, in this case 10. Finally, we can obtain a "cumulative" probability distribution by starting at the lowest score and adding probabilities. This distribution tells you what proportion of the sample fell in and below the category score, thus 6/10 or 60 percent of Hs had scores below 8.6. The concept is best illustrated by the illustration in Figure 9.3, which shows the distributions for the two groups. They start at 0 at the far left, and eventually accumulate up to 1.0 as scores increase to the right.

The Kolmogorov-Smirnov test focuses on the difference between these cumulative probability distributions. If the Ps have, on the average, a lower score than the Hs, then their cumulative distribution will rise to 10/10 more rapidly, as is the case in our data. The greater the difference between scores on the average, the greater will be the difference between the two cumulative distributions in any category.

Now the good news: No fancy calculations or formulas are required to do the Kolmogorov-Smirnov test. All you do is subtract the two probabilities in each category to determine the difference between the two distributions, then find the category with the maximum difference. In our data, that occurs from 6.5 to 8.5, a difference of 3/10 or 0.3. That is the value of the Kolmogorov-Smirnov test. And you look it up in yet another table and find out that the critical value is 0.6, so the difference is not significant.

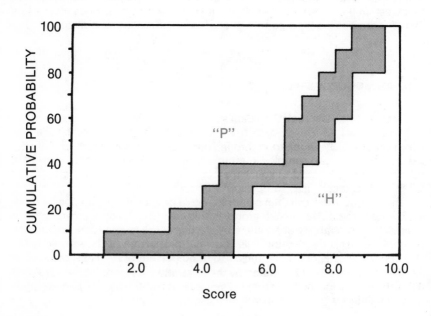

Figure 9.3 Cumulative probability distributions of 'H' and 'P' groups

TESTS OF ORDINAL VARIABLES ON MATCHED SAMPLES

All of the preceding tests on ordinal variables were based on differences among two or more independent samples from a population equivalent to an unpaired t test in parametric statistics. We have not dealt with the matched or paired situation as yet.

As an example on which to display our wares, suppose a social psychologist predicts that height, since it is one feature of dominance and power, is likely to be associated with success in life. (Before we proceed, we should inform you that one of us is 6'5" tall.) In order to cancel out the effect of other environmental variables, such as parents' social class which might lead, on the one hand to better nutrition and greater height, and on the other to an "inherited" higher class, the investigator chooses twins of the same sex as subjects. He follows them into adulthood, and determines the socioeconomic status (a combination of job class, income, educational level) of the taller and shorter twin.

Suppose the researcher could only locate 10 twins (research grants are hard to come by in the social sciences). The data might look like:

Table 9.4A   Sign Test for Correlation of Height and Socioeconomic Status in Twins of the Same Sex

Pair	Taller Twin	Shorter Twin	Difference	Direction
a	87	65	22	+
b	44	40	4	+
c	55	46	9	+
d	69	58	11	+
e	29	16	13	+
f	52	55	−3	−
g	77	60	17	+
h	35	40	−5	−
i	68	50	18	+
j	13	15	−2	−

THE SIGN TEST

The sign test, not surprisingly, focuses on the signs of the differences. If there is no association between height and social status, you would expect that, on the average, half the signs would be + and half −. The statistical question is, "What is the likelihood that a 7/3 split could occur by chance?" Having reduced the situation to a simple difference between pluses and minuses, the approach is identical to the computational approach we outlined in the Binomial test: You calculate the probability of 7 pluses and 3 minuses, 8 and 2, 9 and 1, and 10 and 0. As it turns out, the probability of obtaining a 7/3 split of pluses and minuses is 0.172, which is not significant.

THE WILCOXON TEST

The problem with the sign test, when it is used for ordinal data, is that it ignores the magnitude of the differences. The Wilcoxon test is a bit better in this respect. Let's go back to the data and order it by the magnitude of these differences.

Table 9.4B   Wilcoxon Test for Correlation of Height and Socioeconomic Status in Twins of the Same Sex

Pair	Difference	Rank (+)	Rank (−)
a	22	10	
i	18	9	
g	17	8	
e	13	7	
d	11	6	
c	9	5	
h	−5		4
b	4	3	
f	−3		2
j	−2		1
			7

We're still not allowed to put any direct interpretation on the actual magnitude of the differences, but we can at least say that a difference of 22 is larger than a difference of 18, so the rank ordering of differences has some significance. If there were no relationship between height and status, we would expect that the positive and negative differences would be pretty well intermixed in ranking, and the average rank of positive and negative differences should be about the same.

The Wilcoxon test focuses on these differences in ranks by simply summing the ranks of one sign or another, whichever is ranked lower. In this case, the sum is 7, and if this is located in the appropriate table, the difference is significant at the 0.02 level.

If we blindly assumed that socioeconomic status was interval, and calculated a paired t test, the t value would be 2.79, significant at the 0.02 level. So it would appear that the Wilcoxon test, which uses the information about the magnitude of the differences, results in little loss of information in comparison with parametric tests. By contrast, the sign test, which reduces the ordinal data to a + or −, results in a more conservative test.

DISCUSSION

That's the cookbook of tests that have been applied to ordinal data to test the differences between a sample and theoretical distribution, two samples, or more than two samples. It won't be a surprise to discover that there are a few more tests we've left off, such as the Mosteller test of slippage, the K-sample runs test, the randomization test, etc., et al., ad nauseum.

With all these choices, it's a little difficult to make specific recommendations concerning which statistical test to apply and under which circumstances. In general, the Mann-Whitney and Kruskal-Wallis tests are more powerful, yielding results that are close to parametric tests, and are therefore preferred.

Example 9.1

A naturopath wishes to examine the effect of red iron oxide (rust) supplements on people with anemia. He takes 20 patients, measures their hemoglobin level and catagorizes the disease as mild (>10 g) and severe (<10 g). Before the study based on clinical information, were 12 mild and 8 severe patients. After the dust settles, there are 16 mild and 4 severe. The investigator does a chi-square on the 2 × 2 table, and writes up his study for publication. There are two boo-boos in the approach, can you spot them?

Answer

First, taking a nice ratio variable such as hemoglobin level and shoving it into two categories is an atrocity. The appropriate test is a paired t test on the differences. Second, these are before–after measurements, so a paired test should be used. If he wanted to categorize, a McNemar test would do. The Wilcoxon would be the right test for ordinal data.

C.R.A.P. **DETECTOR #9.1**

Classifying ordinal or interval data in nominal categories is throwing away information, as we have said many times.

C.R.A.P. **DETECTOR #9.2**

Watch out for small expected frequencies. Exact tests should be used if any expected frequency gets to 5 or therabouts.

C.R.A.P. DETECTOR #9.3

People often forget that they have matched or before-after measurements. In general, using unpaired tests on these data results in conservative tests.

NON-PARAMETRIC MEASURES
OF ASSOCIATION

> Several non-parametric measures of association, equivalent to the correlation coefficient, have been devised. These include the *contingency coefficient*, the *phi coefficient*, and *Cohen's kappa coefficient* for nominal data, and *Spearman's rho, Kendall's tau* and *Kendall's W* for ordinal data.

You will recall in the section on parametric statistics that just about the time we had conquered the complexities of multiple group comparisons and factorial ANOVA, we were hauled up short by the recognition that not all questions can be addressed by throwing folks into groups. At that point we regressed (pun) to a study of correlation and regression, methods to measure the amount of association among two or more interval variables measured in a single sample. When we did this we found that, in addition to determining whether an association was statistically significant, we could also express the strength of the association by a correlation coefficient which ranged between −1 and 1.

In this chapter we will examine a number of ways to achieve the same end for nominal and ordinal data. We are seeking a coefficient which can be used on these data, and which will, ideally, have a value of +1 when there is a perfect relationship between the two variables. A perfect relationship exists when one variable can be predicted exactly from knowledge of the other, −1 when there is a perfect inverse relationship, and 0 when there is no relationship between the two variables.

As usual, things aren't quite so clear cut when you get to non-parametric measures of association. We will discuss three measures applicable to nominal data: The contingency coefficient, the phi coefficient, and Cohen's kappa coefficient. Three other measures require ordinal ranks: The Spearman rank correlation, Kendall's tau coefficient, and another coefficient by the prolific Dr. Kendall, the Kendall W coefficient. As usual, they all give different answers and have different strengths and weaknesses, which we'll point out as we go along.

MEASURES OF ASSOCIATION FOR NOMINAL VARIABLES

At first glance, anyone steeped in the tradition of correlation coefficients might view the idea of a measure of association for nominal variables as somewhat preposterous. After all, when you calculate a correlation coefficient, you are measuring the degree to which someone who is high or low on one variable will be high or low on another. Nominal variables are completely egalitarian and unprejudiced: No one is higher or lower than anyone else, they are just different. But the idea of association for nominal variables is not that ridiculous. For nominal variables, the idea of association relates to frequencies in categories. Since most men have beards, and since relatively few women shave daily, it is a natural conclusion that sex and facial hair are associated, without having to decide whether shaving is higher or lower than not shaving.

To explore the question further, let's focus on that dreaded scourge of mankind, Somaliland camel bite fever. Fortunately, we are no longer devastated by this disease thanks to a dedicated investigator who discovered that the serum sage level can diagnose the early stages of the disease so that treatment can be implemented. How reliable is the test? Suppose we had test results for 100 patients being treated for fever and 100 controls, and that the sage test has two values—ripe and raw. The results are displayed in Table 10.1.

Table 10.1   Comparison of Serum Sage Levels in Controls and Patients with Somaliland Camel Bite Fever

Test Result	Patients	Controls	Totals
Ripe	80	30	110
Raw	20	70	90
Total	100	100	200

It certainly looks like there is an association between a positive test result and the scourge: 80 percent of patients versus 30 percent of normals have a ripe sage. If we wanted to test whether the association is statistically significant (i.e., different from zero) we could calculate a chi-square, which turns out to be equal to 50.51 and is highly significant.

THE CONTINGENCY COEFFICIENT

However, the question we are addressing in this chapter is not whether the association is present or absent, but whether there is some way to develop standard measures of the degree of association in order to compare one set of variables to another. The simplest measure is the contingency coefficient, which is based directly on the calculated X^2. It is calculated as:

$$C = \sqrt{\frac{X^2}{(N + X^2)}}$$

where N is the sample size. In this case, the contingency coefficient is equal to

$$C = \sqrt{\frac{50.5}{200 + 50.5}} = 0.45$$

The coeffecient seems to do some of the right things: The larger X^2 is, the closer the value will be to one, and it has the virtue of being easy to calculate. Unfortunately, the beast has one undesirable property, namely it doesn't go to 1 when there is a perfect relationship. In the present example, if the sage test were perfect, chi-square would equal 200, and the coefficient would equal 0.707.

THE PHI COEFFICIENT

This coefficient is a ratio of two quantities, determined as follows. We label the 4 cells in a contingency table a, b, c, and d, by convention, as in Table 10.2.

Table 10.2   Contingency Table Depicting Ratios

	Disease Present	Disease Absent	Totals
Positive	a	b	a + b
Negative	c	d	c + d
Totals	a + c	b + d	N

If there is no association between test and disease, the two ratios a/b and c/d would be equal, and equal to the proportion of people in the sample with the disease. So the ratio of these two numbers would be 1, and if we subtract one from this ratio of ratios, we end up with a number related to the degree of association between the two variables. Playing around a bit with the algebra we have:

$$\frac{(a/b)}{(c/d)} - 1 = \frac{(ad - bc)}{bc}$$

Actually, the phi coefficient uses a different denominator made up of the product of the marginals:

$$\phi = \frac{ad - bc}{\sqrt{(a + b)(c + d)(a + c)(b + d)}} = \frac{80 \times 70 - 20 \times 30}{\sqrt{110 \times 90 \times 100 \times 100}} = 0.50$$

If there is strong association, b and c equal zero, so phi becomes

$$\phi = \frac{ad}{\sqrt{a \times d \times a \times d}} = 1.$$

And if there is no association, ad = bc, and ϕ equals 0. So it looks like phi does the right thing at the extremes.

COHEN'S KAPPA

There is one other simple measure of association that deserves a bit of mention. The upper left cell in a contingency table—positive test, disease present—and the bottom right cell—negative test, disease absent—are cells where there is agreement between test and standard. One simple way to look at association would be to ask what proportion of cases result in agreement, in this case

$$\frac{(80 + 70)}{200} = 0.75. \text{ No statistics required.}$$

Unfortunately, this simple approach has serious problems. Certainly the upper limit is okay. If there is perfect association, all the cases will be in these two cells. But if there is no association at all, there would be

$$\frac{(110 \times 100)}{200} = 55$$

cases in the top left and

$$\frac{(90 \times 100)}{200} = 45$$

cases in the bottom right cell, and the agreement equals

$$\frac{(55 + 45)}{200} = 0.50.$$

Dr. Cohen started from the notion of agreement on the diagonal cells as a measure of association, but corrected for chance agreement. In our example, the actual agreement was 0.75, and chance agreement, as calculated above, was 0.5.

The formula for Kappa is:

$$K = \frac{\text{observed agreement - chance agreement}}{1 - \text{chance agreement}}$$

So in this example,

$$K = \frac{(0.75 - 0.5)}{(1.0 - 0.5)} = 0.50$$

If there is a perfect association observed agreement = 1 and Kappa = 1. No association puts the observed agreement equal to chance agreement and Kappa = 0.

These desirable properties make Kappa the measure of choice for nominal data and 2×2 tables. But all of the coefficients have problems when the number of categories are increased and the data are ordinal. Which, of course, bring us to the coefficients designed for use on ordinal data.

MEASURES OF ASSOCIATION FOR ORDINAL VARIABLES

SPEARMAN RANK CORRELATION COEFFICIENT (RHO)

Time for another example. Our colleagues in rheumatology have devised, at last count, about 30 ways to tell how sick a patient with rheumatoid arthritis is. They range from the sublime—serum this and that levels, to the ridiculous—

how long it takes to stagger the 100 yard dash. Unfortunately, the relationship among all these measures is a bit underwhelming. Let's look at two old favorites: Joint Counts, as the name implies, is a count of the number of inflamed joints, and Clinician Ratings is a test that gives clinical judgment its due. Joint Count is a ratio variable, but frequently they rate each joint on a 3-point scale, which makes it more ordinal. The ratings are on a 10-point scale. The data for eight patients are displayed in Table 10.3.

Table 10.3   Comparison of Joint Count and Clinician Rating in the Assessment of Polyarthritis

Patient	Joint Count	Rank	Clinician Rating	Rank
A	85	2	9	1
B	20	6	3.5	5
C	60	4	6	3
D	25	5	1	8
E	95	1	8	2
F	70	3	5	4
G	10	8	2	7
H	15	7	3	6

You may notice that in good non-parametric style we determined the ranks of each patient on JC and CR in addition to the absolute number. We could go ahead and calculate a Pearson correlation on the original data, but a quick look at the data shows that the numbers are hardly normally distributed, and they are ordinal in any case. So there is good justification to go the non-parametric route.

The basis of the Spearman correlation is the difference in ranks of each pair. If the two variables were perfectly correlated the patient ranked highest on JC would also be highest on CR. In other words, there would be a perfect correspondence in ranks of each patient on the two variables: 1–1, 2–2, and on down to 8–8. The difference in ranks for each pair would all be zero. Conversely, if there were a perfect inverse relationship, the ranked pairs would look like 1–8, 2–7, 3–6, ... 8–1.

Spearman, in deriving the formula that won him international acclaim, began with the formula for the product-moment correlation, but proceeded to calculate the correlation for pairs of ranks, rather than raw data. We won't bore you with the details, but it turns out that some simplifications emerge. In the end, the equivalent formula to the Pearson correlation for ranked data becomes:

$$R_s = 1 - \frac{6 \times (\text{Sum of } d^2)}{N^3 - N}$$

where d is the difference in ranks on the two variables, and N is the number of people. In our example, R_s turns out to be 0.81.

More generally, it is evident that if the data were perfectly correlated, each d would be 0, and the correlation would equal 1. If the data were inversely correlated, it turns out that the correlation is −1. So Spearman's little gem has the desirable characteristic that it has appropriate upper and lower limits. But although it is derived directly from the product–moment correlation, when the distributions really are normal, it is only 91 percent as efficient as the Pearson correlation.

KENDALL'S TAU

Kendall's Tau is used under the same circumstances as the Spearman correlation. Of course, the approach is different. It has the dubious advantage that it requires no algebra, only counts. It has the disadvantage that it yields a different and lower answer than Spearman using the same data, although it is preferred when there are a lot of tied ranks.

So here we go again. The data from our study have been rearranged slightly so JC ranks are in ascending order.

				Patient				
Test	E	A	F	C	D	B	H	G
Joint Count	1	2	3	4	5	6	7	8
Clinical Rating	2	1	4	3	8	5	6	7

Having ordered the JC ranks, the question is, "How many of the possible pairs of CR ranks are in the right order?" A pairwise comparison is done, with +1 assigned to pairs that are in the right order, and −1 to pairs that aren't. If there was a perfect relationship every pair would be assigned a +1, so there would be as many +1s as there are pairs.

This is how it works in the example:

2−1, 2−4, 2−3, 2−8, 2−5, 2−6, 2−7, 1−4, 1−3, 1−8, 1−5, 1−6, 1−7, 4−3,
−1,   +1,   +1,   +1,   +1,   +1,   +1,   +1,   +1,   +1,   +1,   +1,   +1,   −1

4−8, 4−5, 4−6, 4−7, 3−8, 3−5, 3−6, 3−7, 8−5, 8−7, 5−6, 5−7, 6−7
+1,   +1,   +1,   +1,   +1,   +1,   +1,   +1,   −1,   −1,   +1,   −1,   −1

The +s and −s are then summed, to $23-5 = 18$. This sum is divided by the maximum possible score which is $N(N-1)/2 = 28$, (i.e., the number of pairs). So for these data, tau is equal to $18/28 = 0.64$, which you may note compares to 0.81 for the Spearman coefficient. This is perhaps not surprising since the coefficient, like the Sign test, uses only the direction and not the magnitude of the differences. Although it is conservative, it is better when there are many tied ranks. However tau is restricted to only two groups. Perhaps that's why Dr. Kendall invented another coefficient...

KENDALL'S W (COEFFICIENT OF CONCORDANCE)

One problem shared by all the coefficients discussed so far is that, like the standard Pearson correlation, they can only consider the association between two variables at a time. The occasion may arise when one might wish to say what is the agreement overall among several variables. The situation often emerges in examining the agreement among multiple raters or the association among more than two variables.

Suppose a researcher wanted to obtain ratings of the interpersonal skills of a group of physical therapy students from patients, supervisors, and peers. The question now is the extent of agreement among the 3 ratings of each student. Using 6 therapists, suppose their ratings on a scale ended up ranked like this:

Student	Patient	Supervisor	Student	Sum of Ranks
A	1	2	3	6
B	2	1	1	4
C	3	3	2	8
D	4	6	4	14
E	5	4	6	15
F	6	5	5	16

In the righthand column we have taken the liberty of summing the ranks for each therapist. If there were perfect agreement among the observers, then therapist A would be ranked 1st by everyone, and therapist F last by all, so then summed rank for A would be $1 \times$ (number of observers), in this case 3, and for F would be (number of therapists) $\times$ (number of observers) $= 6 \times 3 = 18$. By contrast, if there is no association, then every summed rank would end up about the same. So one measure of the degree of association would be to determine the difference between individual rank sums and the mean rank sum. Of course, statisticians have a reflex response to square every difference they encounter, and this case is no exception. The starting point in calculating Kendall's W is to determine the summed rank for each case, and the average summed rank, take the difference for each case, and add up the square of all the differences.

In our example, the average summed rank is

$$\frac{(6 + 4 + 8 + 14 + 15 + 16)}{6} = 10.5$$

So the sum of the squared deviations is

$$(6 - 10.5)^2 + (4 - 10.5)^2 + (8 - 10.5)^2 + \ldots (16 - 10.5)^2 = 131.5$$

Now the next challenge is to figure out the maximum value that this sum of squares could achieve. A little algebra (trust us) demonstrates that this is equal to

$$\frac{1 \ (3)^2 \ (6^3 - 6)}{12} = \frac{1 \ (9)(216 - 6)}{12} = 157.5$$

So the coefficient of association now is simply the ratio of the actual sum of squared differences to the maximum possible (i.e., $131.5/157.5 = 0.83$). And that's that! By the way, application of this formula to the data used for the Spearman correlation yields a value of 0.91, versus 0.81 for R_s and 0.64 for tau.

That about brings us to the end of the potpourri of measures of association and agreement. Focusing on the measures applied to ordinal data, Spearman's rho coefficient is far and away the winner of the popularity poll in terms of actual usage. Kendall's W is very similar, and has the advantage that it can be used as a measure of association for multiple observations. Kendall's T is a little different and has three advantages: it is a little easier to calculate, it is better for tied ranks, and it can be used to calculate partial correlations, an area we didn't touch on. But it gives considerably lower answers in general than the previous two coefficients.

Example 10.1

Suppose we choose to look at inter-rater agreement of back mobility judgments by chiropracters. Two methods are advocated - direct estimation of range of motion in degrees and clinician ratings of hypermobile, normal range, and restricted range. What coefficients would you use? Any guesses as to which would be larger?

Answer

Since range of motion in degrees is ratio, a Pearson correlation would be best. However, if more than two raters are involved, Kendall's W would give a good overall picture of rater agreement. You might use Kappa for clinician ratings, but these are actually crude ordinal data, so a coefficient based on ranks would be better. The loss of information in the 3-point scale implies that the Kappa would be lower.

C.R.A.P. DETECTOR #10.1

If the data are reasonably interval and normal, as with many rating scales, a Pearson correlation is best.

C.R.A.P. DETECTOR #10.2

A similar argument holds within non-parametric domain. Measures for nominal data like Kappa will give low values when applied to ordinal data in comparison to the appropriate ordinal measures.

C.R.A.P. **DETECTOR #10.3**

People often use multiple raters and then calculate
agreement between 1 and 2, 1 and 3, 7 and 8, and so
on. Generally, any differences among rater pairs
usually reflects statistical variation, and an overall
measure of agreement such as Kendall's W is much
preferred.

ADVANCED NON-PARAMETRIC METHODS

> There are three approaches to handling designs
> where the dependent variable involves frequencies in
> categories, with more than one independent variable.
> *Mantel-Haenzel chi-square* deals with two indepen-
> dent factors. Logistic regression and log-linear anal-
> ysis can handle any number of independent variables.
> *Logistic regression* treats all independent variables
> as measured data like multiple regression. *Log-linear
> analysis* handles the case of multiple categorical vari-
> ables, and estimates effects and interactions, analo-
> gous to factorial ANOVA.

On reflection you may realize that something is missing from the preceding
two chapters. None of the methods we considered goes beyond the equivalent
of one-way ANOVA or simple correlations; they all consider only two variables
at a time.

Naturally this void hasn't escaped the notice of statisticians. Several methods
have been developed to deal with the relation among multiple independent
variables and a counted dependent variable. The Mantel-Haenzel chi-square
handles two categorical independent variables. Logistic regression is an extension of multiple regression approaches to handle nominal dependent variables.
Finally, log-linear analysis estimates frequencies where there are multiple categorical independent variables.

MANTEL-HAENZEL CHI-SQUARE

The simplest clinical trial involves randomly assigning patients to one of two
categories, such as drug or placebo, or treatment A versus treatment B. An outcome event such as death or relapse is then counted in each group, and the
frequencies are compared using a chi-square test.

One common refinement of this approach is called prognostic stratification.
If, for example, age is likely to be associated with the outcome event (i.e., old
folks are more likely to die during the course of the study), then the sample
is stratified to ensure that equal numbers of folks in each age group end up
in the two groups. It is still legitimate simply to compare event rates in the two
large groups, but it is also desirable to examine events in each age subgroup
to test whether treatment effects are consistent across all ages.

A similar situation arises in studies of risk factors for disease. Having demon-strated, by assembling a series of patients who got the disease and controls who didn't, that patients are more likely to have been exposed to a particular noxious agent, we might want to show that the effect is consistent across all age and sex subgroups.

As an example, suppose we want to examine the relationship between the punker practice of inserting safety pins in earlobes and noses and hepatitis B. Since other practices in this subculture, such as using injectable drugs, might also lead to a higher rate of hepatitis, we may wish to stratify by drug use: none, moderate, and heavy use.

We assemble a few hundred punkers with hepatitis who checked into the Liverpool General, locate a comparable group of relatively healthy punkers, and inquire about safety pin and drug use. The data are arrayed in Table 11.1.

Table 11.1　Association of Hepatitis B Among Drug Users and Pin Users

Drug Use	Pin Use	Hepatitis B		Total
		Yes	No	
None	Yes	78	40	220
	No	27	75	
Moderate	Yes	92	29	174
	No	19	34	
Heavy	Yes	60	209	454
	No	5	180	
Total		281	567	848

By inspection, there certainly appears to be an association between safety pins and hepatitis B. But there is also a relation between pin use and drug use: 54 percent of non-drug users use pins, compared to 72 percent of heavy drug users also using pins. Because both drug use and pin use are associated with hepatitis B, simply adding the subtables together to calculate an overall chi-square is going to underestimate the effect. It's a bit like the situation in analy-sis of covariance. Some of the variance in the event rates can be attributed to the use of drugs, so controlling for the effect of this variable will improve the likelihood of detecting a difference due to the primary variable of interest, safety pins.

So how do you analyze across subtables without committing the ultimate atrocity of repeated statistical tests? Mantel and Haenzel began with the origi-nal definition of chi-square, as we did in Chapter 9. If we focus on the upper left cell in each table (labelled "a" by convention), it's easy to figure out the expected value of "a" if there were no association between pins and hepatitis. For the "no drug" group, this is just:

$$\text{Expected Value} = \frac{(a + b) \times (a + c)}{N} = \frac{118 \times 105}{220} = 56.3$$

The variance of this estimate is another product of marginals:

$$\text{Variance} = \frac{(a + b)(a + c)(b + d)(c + d)}{N^2 (N - 1)} = \frac{105 \times 115 \times 102 \times 118}{(220 \times 220 \times 219)} = 13.7$$

This step can be repeated for all the subtables. The final bit of subterfuge results from adding up all the a's. If there was no association, the sum of the a's should be normally distributed with a mean equal to the sum of the expected values and a variance equal to the sum of the variances. So the quantity

$$\text{Chi-square} = \frac{(\text{sum of a's} - \text{sum of expected a's})^2}{\text{sum of variances}}$$

is a chi-square, which can be associated with a probability in the usual way. This is the overall test of the association between safety pins and hepatitis B, and turns out to equal 74.2, a highly significant association. If we had just gone ahead and calculated a chi-square based on the summary table over all levels of drug use, the result would be 55.9. So by controlling for drug use we have improved the sensitivity of the test.

The Mantel-Haenzel chi-square is, in a sense, the non-parametric equivalent of using a covariate in analysis of covariance. It can be used to correct for bias caused by different numbers of cases in the subgroups, to improve sensitivity of the overall test as we demonstrated above, and to investigate interactions between the two factors (i.e., "Is the effect of safety pins different across the levels of drug use?").

However, the Mantel-Haenzel chi-square is limited to only two independent variables. Two other methods are available to handle multiple independent variables, namely logistic regression and log-linear analysis.

Before we get to these multivariate methods, there is one special application of the Mantel-Haenzel procedure which deserves further mention. A very common situation in clinical trials, particularly those in which the variable of interest is death, is that people don't wait until the last day of the study to die. This forces researchers to construct a life table, and invoke special methods for analysis.

LIFE TABLE ANALYSIS

In most of the studies described so far, the end point occurs at some fairly definite point, which is often under the control of the researcher, e.g., responses to two drugs are measured a few hours or weeks after administration; demographic and clinical or performance data are gathered at entry and exit from a program, and so forth. Some studies, though, are not as neat, and the outcome appears in its own sweet time. A prime example of this would be cancer trials, where the outcome, usually death, can occur within days after the person is entered into the trial, or may not happen until many years have passed. Indeed, our interest is in how long it takes to reach this end point ("Sir, I regret to inform you that your father has reached his end point!")

However, there are at least three methodological problems which require the use of a different form of analysis, usually called life table analysis or survival curve analysis. The first difficulty is that patients are usually enrolled into the study over a protracted period of time. In large studies, it would be unusual to have enough diabetic or cancer patients at any one point so that they can all begin the trial on the same day. Having to follow these patients over a long interval (often years) leads to the other two difficulties. During this time, we would lose track of some people because they may move, get tired of the study, or tell us to go fly a kite, and we would have no way of knowing what happens to them. Further, the funding agency may remind us that all good things must come to an end, including our study.

So, at the end of the study, rather than just the one neat end point we anticipated, our subjects have three possible outcomes—deceased (or in relapse, depending on the nature of the trial); lost to follow-up after varying periods of time; and still alive (or well) after varying periods. Complicating the issue a bit more, the "varying periods" can be the result of two different causes: the drop-outs can occur at any time the patient moves or gets fed up; and, since the patients are enrolled over the course of the study, they are at risk for different periods at the point when we stop the study. These different possibilities are shown in Figure 11.1, where a W indicates withdrawal, and X means the subject died.

Subjects 1, 4, 9, and 10 died during the trial; numbers 3, 6, and 7 withdrew; while Subjects 2, 5, and 8 were still alive when the study ended in Year 5. (The data from these last three people are referred to as "censored." This simply means that the study ended before they did, and casts no aspersions on their moral virtues.) The question we now have to answer is, "How long do patients survive after they begin treatment?" If we base our conclusions only on the subjects for whom we have complete data, then it would be the mean of 30 months (Subject 1), 10 months (Subject 4), 14 months (Subject 9), and 16 months (Subject 10), or just under 1½ years. This approach is unsatisfying for two reasons: we've discarded much of our data, and we haven't taken into account that the surviving subjects are indeed still around and kicking when we had to end the study. Also, what do we do with the withdrawals? Obviously, we can't determine length of survival from their data, but they did provide useful information before they withdrew.

We can get around some of these problems in a way dear to a researcher's heart: if we don't like the answer, let's change the question. What we *can* look at is the proportion of people who were still alive at the end of 1 year; the proportion alive at the end of 2 years if they were in the study at the end of 1 year, and so on. To make our job easier, let's redraw Figure 11.1 so that it looks like everyone started at the same time. This yields Figure 11.2, where W and X have the same meaning as before, and A indicates that the person was alive when the study ended.

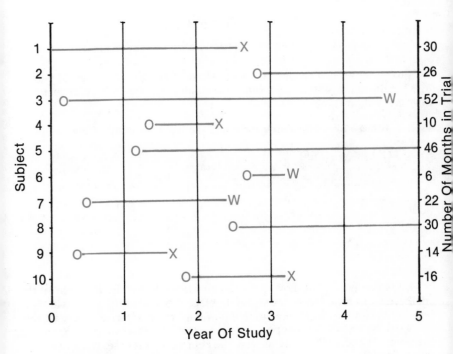

Figure 11.1   Entry and withdrawal of subjects in a 5-year study

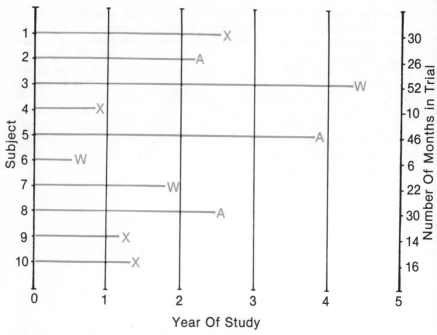

Figure 11.2   Putting all subjects at a common starting point

From this we can easily make a life table showing the number of people in the study at the start of each year, how many withdrew during that year, and how many died (Table 11.2).

Table 11.2   Life Table for the E. Ternal Longevity Study

Years in Study	Number of Patients at Risk	Number of Deaths in Year	Withdrawals During the Year
0 - 1	10	1	1
1 - 2	8	2	1
2 - 3	5	1	2
3 - 4	2	0	1
4 - 5	1	0	1

So far, so good. But, how many patients died during the first year of the trial? We know for a fact that one did, Subject 4, but what do we do with Subject 6? He withdrew some time during the year—we're not sure exactly when—but we don't know what happened to him. Here we make an assumption that the person withdrew half-way through the interval, in this case, 1 year. Actually, this is less of a leap of faith than it seems. If the trial is large enough, and if withdrawals occur at random, then this would simply be the mean time that these subjects are at risk.

During the first year, then, 9½ people were at risk of dying—9 people for one year, and 1 person for half a year—of whom 1 actually died. So, the risk of dying during the first year is 1/9.5, or 0.1053. Conversely, the probability of surviving is 1 - 0.1053, or 0.8947. Similarly, during Year 2, 7.5 people were at risk, of whom 2 died, so the probability of surviving the second year *if you were around when the year began*, is 0.7333. The chances of surviving the entire 2-year span is the probability of making it through the first year (0.8947) times the probability of living through the interval between Years 1 and 2 (0.7333), or 0.6561.

Five people entered the third year of the trial, but 2 withdrew. Crediting each as being at risk for half a year, we have 1 death in 4 person-years, for a probability of surviving of 0.75. Thus, the chances of surviving all three years is 0.6561 × 0.75, or 0.4921. In our admittedly sparse trial, no deaths occurred during the last 2 years, so the probabilities don't change. If we now plot the cumulative probabilities for each year, as in Figure 11.3, we'll have our survival curve.

Although we can get much useful information from this type of life table analysis, its real glory comes when we *compare* two treatments, or a treatment versus a control, and so on. We start out exactly the same way, deriving a life table for each condition. Our questions now are: (1) "At any given point in the trial, is one arm doing better than the other?" and (2) "At the end of the trial, are there better overall results from one condition as compared with the other?" Although the computations are a bit more complex than we'd like to get into, especially in figuring out the standard error, the technique boils down in both cases to a Mantel-Haenzel chi-square, which we've just discussed.

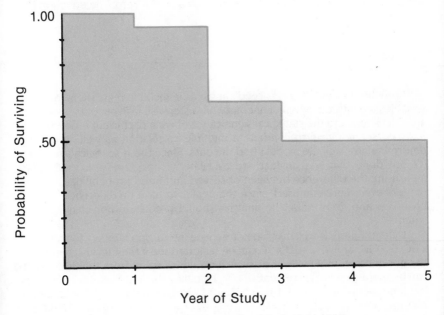

Figure 11.3   Survival curve for data in Table 11.2

LOGISTIC REGRESSION

In Chapter 5, we reviewed a technique, multiple regression, which was specifically designed to predict a single dependent variable using a number of independent variables. The trouble with using the method in the present situation is that our dependent variable has only two values: alive or dead, diseased or healthy, 0 or 1. To treat something with only two values as a sample from a normal distribution requires a leap of faith which even statisticians aren't prepared to make. However, by a simple transformation, called a logistic function or logit, we can make the variable look a lot more reasonable. That is the essence of logistic regression.

As an example, suppose we are attempting to determine which of a group of women at a fertility clinic are most likely to become pregnant. Some factors which may influence the happy event are age (AGE), frequency of intercourse (IC), and father's sperm count (SC), all ratio variables, and prior history of birth control pills (BCP) and IUD use (IUD), both categorical nominal variables.

Forgetting for the moment that pregnancy is the ultimate categorical variable, a multiple regression equation might look like

$$\text{Pregnancy} = a + b_1(\text{AGE}) + b_2(\text{IC}) + b_3(\text{SC}) + b_4(\text{BCP}) + b_5(\text{IUD})$$

where BCP and IUD $= 1$ if there is a history of contraceptive use, and 0 if not.

To make pregnancy act a little more like a regular variable, the next step is to convert it to a logistic function, $\log (p/1-p)$ which is quite well-behaved. For a p of 0.5, it equals 0, and it is symmetrical about zero. The equation then becomes

$$\text{Log} \frac{p}{1 - p} = b_0 + b_1(\text{AGE}) + b_2(\text{IC}) + b_3(\text{SC}) + b_4(\text{BCP}) + b_5(\text{IUD})$$

From here on in, things proceed almost as in multiple regression. Individual variables are introduced simultaneously or in stepwise fashion, beta-coefficients are calculated, and the statistical significance of each coefficient is determined. It would seem logical to compute a multiple correlation as well, in order to determine how well the model fitted the data. Since this is so logical, in general it's not done that way. Instead we calculate a "goodness-of-fit" chi-square, measuring the difference between observed and fitted probabilities. To make matters even more confused, since the goal is to have no difference between observed and fitted data, the analysis should produce a non-significant chi-square.

Different models which include or exclude interaction terms of the form AGE x SC, SC x IC, or AGE x IUD x SC can be tested to see if their inclusion improves the goodness of fit. Finally, the coefficients which result from the fitted model can be converted back to a relative risk, by taking the anti logarithm. For example, if the beta-coefficient for IUD was -0.32, then the odds of pregnancy with IUD use over no IUD use is $\exp(-0.32) = 0.73$. That is to say an IUD user is 27 percent less likely to become pregnant than the non-user of IUDs.

One final comment on the method. As we get to multiple variables, the distinction between categorical and continuous data becomes blurred. In the previous example, we did elegant transformations on the dependent variable to make it "act" like a measurement, but we were quite happy to treat IUD status as just 1 or 0. As you will find in Chapter 14, discriminant function analysis is a form of parametric statistics which treats exactly the problem approached by logistic regression. The approach is different, naturally, but fortunately it seems the two methods yield approximately the same answer.

LOG-LINEAR ANALYSIS

Unlike logistic regression, log-linear analysis is designed to analyze only categorical variables. Further, it does not distinguish between independent and dependent variables; alive/dead is just one more category like over 50/under 50 or male/female. Let's use a relatively simple 3-factor case, the drug use/hepatitis problem which began this chapter. You may wish to have another look at Table 11.1 to refresh your memory.

The basis of the log-linear analysis is a thing called an effect. To see how the idea derives, let's examine what the data would look like if there were no association at all among all the factors. The frequency in each cell would be predicted exactly by the product of the marginals, using the same approach which was first introduced in the chi-square test before.

Bringing in a little algebra, let U_1 be the proportion of non-users in the sample

$$U_1 = \frac{(78 + 40 + 27 + 75)}{848} = 0.259$$

Similarly, we can calculate the proportion of moderate (U_2) and heavy (U_3) users. Then using different marginals, we can also calculate the expected proportions for the safety pin use, S_1 and S_2, and for hepatitis B, H_1 and H_2. Then the expected value of each cell, under the hypothesis of no association, is the total sample size, 848, times the product of the appropriate proportions. So for example, the expected frequency in the moderate use / safety pin / hepatitis cell is:

$$\text{Expected Frequency} = 848 \times (U_2 \times S_1 \times H_1) = 34.5$$

The alternative to no association in this problem is some association, but there are several possible associations which can be considered: between hepatitis and pin use (call it HS), between hepatitis and drug use (HU), drug use and pin use (US), or among all three (HUS). In the most extreme case all may be important, so the frequency in a cell will be predicted from all the two-way and three-way proportions:

$$F_{211} = N \times U_2 \times S_1 \times H_1 \times US_{21} \times UH_{21} \times HS_{11} \times HUS_{121}$$

The situation is analogous to factorial ANOVA, where there can be main effects, two-way, three-way, and four-way interactions, with separate tests of significance for each one.

Now comes the magic act. Up until now numbers aren't logarithmic, and they aren't linear. However, it turns out that the logarithm of a product of terms is just the sum of the logs of the individual terms. If we call the logs of our original terms by a different name, so that $\log U_1 = u_1$, then

$$\log(F_{211}) = n + u_2 + s_1 + h_1 + us_{21} + uh_{21} + hs_{11} + hus_{121}$$

So by taking the log we have created a linear model. This of course causes great delight among statisticians, who can go ahead and calculate coefficients with gay abandon. However, the equation we developed is only one model. We began with the "no association" model, which looks like

$$\log(F_{211}) = n + u_2' + s_1' + h_1'$$

Actually there is a family of models, depending on which associations (or effects) are significant. The usual approach is to proceed in a hierarchical fashion, starting with no association, until an adequate fit is achieved. Fit is measured, as with logistic regression, by an overall goodness-of-fit chi-square, and chi-squares on the individual coefficients. If the no association model fits the data, then there's no reason to proceed. But if it doesn't, then two-way interaction effects are introduced one at a time, then in combination, until an adequate fit is obtained and addition of additional effects does not significantly improve the fit.

The alternative strategy is to start with the full-blown model to get a sense of which coefficients are significant, and then test reduced models based on this information. The computer is indifferent to the strategy, so both approaches should lead to the same point.

So we have pretty well exhausted the possibilities for analyzing a single dependent variable. Both logistic regression and log-linear models handle the possibility of multiple independent variables. Logistic regression treats everything as a measured quantity and turns the analysis into a regression problem. Log-linear analysis treats all variables as categorical, and by using a logarithmic transformation, again turns things into a regression-like problem. Like many complex approaches, these methods can be subject to abuse, as the following example illustrates.

Example 11.1

A multicenter trial was conducted comparing surgical and medical management of angina. Surgical treatment entailed the use of bypass grafts, with an operative mortality of 5 percent. Five hundred patients were enrolled in each group and followed for an average of 1.5 years. At the end, there were 35 deaths in the surgical group and 20 deaths in the medical group. The difference was significant (Chi-square $= 4.33$, $p = 0.05$). Would you choose medical therapy?

Answer

No way. If you exclude perioperative mortality, there were only 10 deaths in the surgical treatment group versus 20 in the medically treated group. Patients were only followed for 1.5 years; probably a longer follow-up period would have favored surgical intervention.

C.R.A.P. DETECTOR #11.1

More errors are committed through failure to use life table analysis than by using it. You should have a good idea of when the deaths occurred, and this is best achieved with a life table.

MULTIVARIATE STATISTICS

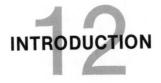

INTRODUCTION

> Around the turn of the century, any charlatan could sell a healing device to a gullible customer simply by saying that it was based on the principles of electricity or magnetism. These fields were in their infancy, and what they did seemed almost magical or miraculous, so that it was difficult for the general public to differentiate between valid and fanciful claims. Being much wiser and more sophisticated now, we would not be taken in by such a sales pitch or fooled by such a fallacious appeal to science. Or would we?

It seems that today's equivalent of electricity is multivariate statistics. It has the aura of science around it, as well as being poorly understood by the uninitiated. It would be unusual to find an article called, "A t test of ...", or "A non-parametric analysis of ...." But we do see many articles which start off, "A multivariate analysis of ...", as though what follows must be truth and beauty. This isn't to say that people who use multivariate statistics are charlatans, but that if multivariate statistics are used, then we often suspend our critical judgment and assume that the conclusions are not only valid, but perhaps even more valid than had univariate statistics been used.

Multivariate statistics do have some advantages and are clearly indicated in some circumstances, but unfortunately, there is also a negative side to this. George Bernard Shaw, in his marvelous play *The Doctor's Dilemma*, had the crusty old physician say, "Chloroform has done a lot of mischief. It's enabled every fool to be a surgeon." In the same way, SPSS and BMDP (two of the most popular sets of "canned" programs) have allowed everybody to be a statistician, whether or not they understand what they are doing, and we have been inundated with highly complex analyses of completely inappropriate data. In this section, we will explore what multivariate statistics are, what their results mean, when they should be used, and when they shouldn't be.

115

WHAT DO WE MEAN BY "MULTIVARIATE"

"Multivariate" means just what it sounds like: many variables. In statistical jargon, it has an even narrower meaning; many dependent variables. (Like the fabled Hungarian nobleman who could only count to three, statisticians call anything more than one, many.) Let's say you want to see if salt-free diets are as effective in reducing hypertension in thin people as in obese individuals. One study could be structured with two groups of men, one at least 25 percent over their ideal body weight, and one at or below ideal weight. Half of each group would be put on a salt-free diet, and the other half would remain on their regular diets. You will measure their diastolic blood pressure (DSP) one month later. This would *not* be considered a multivariate design, since there is only one dependent measure, diastolic blood pressure. The other two variables, weight and diet, are independent variables, so you could stick with a univariate test, such as an analysis of variance.

But, if you wanted to look at both DSP and, say, low density lipoprotein (LDL) cholesterol, you've just graduated to the big time and would have to use one of the multivariate tests. You may wonder why there is this sudden conceptual leap, when all you are doing is measuring a second dependent variable. Why not simply do two or three separate analyses of variance?

There are two major reasons why, both having to do with the fact that any time you measure two or more variables for the same person, those variables are correlated to some degree. Staying with the present example, if you know a person's DSP is 80, you could probably guess his cholesterol level. You won't know the exact level, but you'd be more accurate than if you didn't know his diastolic pressure. Testing each one separately with univariate statistics is a bit unfair. If a significant difference were found between the groups for diastolic pressure, then you would expect to see a difference for LDL cholesterol level, simply because the two are correlated. The two analyses are not independent.

The second reason is almost the obverse of the first. Just as the interaction among independent variables in a factorial ANOVA provides new information, which could not be observed by examining each variable separately, similarly looking at two or more dependent variables simultaneously provides more information than doing a series of separate univariate analyses.

HOTELLING'S T² AND MANOVA

When there is more than one dependent variable, it is inappropriate to do a series of univariate tests. Hotelling T² is used when there are two groups with multiple dependent measures; and MANOVA is used for more than two groups.

HOTELLING'S T² TEST

We'll begin our discussion of specific multivariate tests by taking a look at one called Hotelling's T². To clear up the first mystery, it's called that because it was invented by H. Hotelling, who derived it by taking the equation for Student's t test and squaring it. Basically, it is a t test, modified so that it can be used to look at two or more dependent variables at the same time. Let's return to the example of seeing if salt-reduction has any therapeutic benefit in mildly hypertensive males. To simplify the problem, we'll forget about weight as a factor, and just compare an experimental group on a salt-free diet with a control group. Again, we're interested in two dependent variables; diastolic blood pressure and LDL cholesterol. The data are arrayed in Table 13.1.

Table 13.1   Comparison of Blood Pressure and Serum Cholesterol between Treatment and Control Groups

	Treatment Group	Control Group
Diastolic Blood Pressure		
Mean (mm Hg)	87	95
Standard Deviation	15	21
LDL Cholesterol		
Mean (mmol/L)	2.53	2.09
Standard deviation	0.84	0.79
Sample Size	25	25

Having learned his lessons well, the researcher realizes that he cannot do two separate t tests, since the two measures are most likely correlated with each other to some degree. What he needs is a statistic which will tell him whether the two groups differ on *both* measures when they are looked at simultaneously.

When we looked at Student's t test, we compared the mean of the treatment group with the mean of the control group and tested whether this difference between the groups was greater than the variability of scores within the groups. Now we compare the vector of means in the treatment group with the vector of means in the control group. A vector, in statistical terms, can be thought of simply as a list of values. Here, each vector has two values: the mean for the DSP (the first number in the brackets) and the mean LDL cholesterol level (the second number):

$$x_t = (87, 2.53) \qquad x_c = (95, 2.09)$$

We are not limited to two means per group; the T^2 procedure can handle any number of dependent variables. If the researcher had also measured the serum aldosterone level, then he could still use Hotelling's T^2, and the vector for each group would then consist of three values.

In Figure 13.1, we have plotted what the data might look like, with cholesterol on one axis and DBP on the other. The center of each ellipse is shown as C_t for the treatment group and C_c for the control group. Actually, C_t is plotted at the point where the mean values of cholesterol and DBP intersect for the control group, and similarly for C_c. Statisticians of course like obscure words, and these points are called the centroids of the groups.

The distance between the two means is obvious: Just connect the two centroids and measure the length of the line. This can also be done algebraically as Euclid demonstrated 2,000 years ago. The algebra naturally covers more than two variables, even if graph paper doesn't; it's just a matter of connecting two points in 3-, 4-, or n-dimensional space.

Now let's get back to our original question: "Do these two points (or "centroids" or "vectors of means") differ from each other?" The answer is, we still don't know. As in the case of Student's t test, we have to know a bit more about the data. In the univariate test, this information consists of the variance or standard deviation of the data. In the multivariate case, we need this too, plus one other bit of information, the correlation between (or among) the variables.

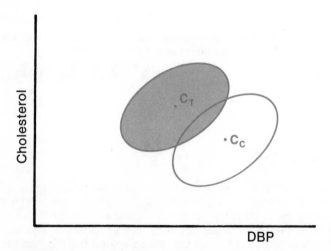

Figure 13.1   Diastolic blood pressure and cholesterol in treatment and control groups

Armed with the wisdom of the variability of scores gleaned from the previous chapters, the reasons for including the variance are self-evident to you. But, you may wonder why we've brought in the correlation coefficient, almost as if from left field.

Let's go back to Figure 13.1. The size and shape of the ellipses tell us that the two variables are correlated positively with one another. That is, a high value on DSP is usually associated with a high value for cholesterol, and vice versa. We can take one of the groups, say the treatment group, as the standard, and look at where the centroid for the other group falls. Notice that the mean value for diastolic blood pressure is *higher* in the control group than in the treatment group; but the mean value for cholesterol is *lower*. That is, the relationship between the two centroids is opposite to that of the variables as a whole—a higher mean on one variable is paired with a lower mean on the other. That would make this finding unusual, at least on an intuitive basis. So, the correlation coefficient tells us that the two variables should be *positively* correlated, and the negative correlation between the two reflects a deviation from the overall pattern.

If the two variables had been *negatively* correlated, on the other hand, we wouldn't make too much of the relationship between the centroids; it simply goes along with what the data as a whole look like.

At this point, let's assume that we've found a significant value of T². What does all this tell us? It means that the *centroids* of the two groups are significantly different from each other. But, there are three ways in which the groups can differ: (1) they can be significantly different on variable 1, but not on variable 2; (2) they can differ on the second variable, but not the first; and (3) both variables may be significantly different. If there were three variables, then there would be seven possible ways the groups could differ; four variables would lead to 15 different ways, and so on. This test does not tell us *which* of these possibilities is actually the case, simply that *one* of them resulted in a significant value of T². In this way, it is analogous to a significant omnibus F ratio. At least two of the groups differ, but we don't know which two. In order to find out, we would have to follow the T² with a different test, such as a multiple discriminant function analysis, which we'll discuss later.

MULTIVARIATE ANALYSIS OF VARIANCE (MANOVA)

So far, we've limited our example to include any number of dependent variables, but only two groups. How would we handle a situation involving more than two groups, as would be the case if we also divided each of the two groups on the basis of their weight? Again, we can use Student's t test as a model. When we wanted to develop the t test to include more than two groups, we derived the analysis of variance (ANOVA). In the same way, we can develop Hotelling's T² to handle more than two groups by expanding it; in this case into what we call a Multivariate Analysis of Variance (MANOVA). The relationship among these four tests is shown in Table 13.2.

Table 13.2   Choice of Analytical Method by Number of Groups and Variables

No. of Dependent Variables	1 or 2 Groups	3 or more Groups
1	t test	ANOVA
2	T^2	MANOVA

If we did an ANOVA on only two groups, the result would be comparable to having calculated t directly. In the exact same way, a MANOVA done on two groups would yield results identical with those of a T^2.

Again, we can get an intuitive grasp of what MANOVA does by beginning with an equivalent univariate statistic, which this table shows to be an ANOVA. In ANOVA, we use an F ratio to determine if the groups are significantly different from each other, and the formula for this test is:

$$F = \frac{\text{Mean Square (treatments)}}{\text{Mean Square (error)}}$$

That is, we are testing whether there is greater variability *between* the groups (i.e., the Treatments effect) than *within* the groups (i.e., Error).

In the case of MANOVA, though, we do not have just one term for the "Treatments" effect and one for the "Error." Rather, we have a *number* of treatment effects and a *number* of error terms. This is due to the fact that, in an ANOVA, each group mean could be represented by a single number; while in a MANOVA, each group has a vector of means, one mean for each variable. So, when we want to examine how much each group differs from the "mean" of all the groups combined, we are really comparing the centroid of each group versus the grand centroid. Similarly, the within-group variability has to be computed for each of the dependent variables.

Again we calculate a ratio, but in this case we have to divide one series of scores by another group of scores. The techniques of how this is done are referred to as matrix algebra and are far beyond the scope of this book. Fortunately, though, there are many computer programs which can do this scut work for us.

However, there are two points which make our life somewhat difficult. First, we have gotten used to the idea that the larger the result of a statistical test, the more significant the findings. For some reason that surpasseth human understanding, this has been reversed in the case of MANOVA. Instead of calculating the Treatments mean square divided by the Error mean square, MANOVA computes the equivalent of the error term divided by the treatment term. Hence, the *smaller* this value is, the more significant the results.

The second problem, which is common to many multivariate procedures, is that we are blessed (or cursed, depending on your viewpoint) with a multitude of different ways to accomplish the same end. In MANOVA, there are many test statistics used to determine if the results are significant. The most widely used method is called Wilk's lambda test, but there are many other procedures which can be used. Arguments about which is the best one to use make the debates among the medieval Scholasticists look tame and restrained. Each method has its believers, and each has its detractors. In most instances, the statistics yield equivalent results. However, if the data are only marginally significant, it's possible that one of the test statistics would tell one thing and the other tests would say the opposite. Then it becomes almost a toss-up which one to believe.

As with the Hotelling T^2 test, a significant finding tells us only that a difference exists *somewhere* in the data, but it doesn't tell us where. For this, we'll again use a discriminant function, explained in the next chapter.

Example 13.1

Our intrepid psoriasis researcher feels that patients who keep kosher may respond differently to clam juice than other people, and so divides each group on this variable.

Question 1

What statistical procedure should he use to see if this factor affects the extent of lesion?

Answer

He would still use a univariate test, like the t test. Kosher versus traif (i.e., non-Kosher) is an independent variable, so there is still only one dependent variable, namely lesion extent.

C.R.A.P. DETECTOR #13.1

Multivariate procedures are used only when there are multiple *dependent* variables, not independent ones.

Question 2

What would happen if he ran a Hotelling T^2 test or MANOVA on the data?

Answer

Although the test statistic will be different (a Wilk's lambda test or F test as opposed to a t test), the conclusions will be the same, since T^2 is a special case of MANOVA (using only two groups), and t is a special case of T^2 (only one dependent variable).

C.R.A.P. **DETECTOR #13.2**

Beware the unneeded multivariate test! It may look more impressive, but if there's only one dependent variable, then the authors are going in for a bit of statistical overkill.

Question 3

Assume he found a significant difference between kosher versus traif. Does this mean that this factor plays a role?

Answer

Not necessarily. In all multivariate procedures, the rule of thumb is that there should be at least 10 subjects per variable. With a smaller subject-to-variable ratio, any result, significant or not, is likely to be unreliable, and probably wouldn't be found if the study were replicated.

C.R.A.P. **DETECTOR #13.3**

Don't regard too seriously any study that used fewer than 10 subjects for each variable.

DISCRIMINANT FUNCTION ANALYSIS

> When there are many dependent variables, significant differences among the groups can be due to the effect of just one variable, some of them, or all of them. *Discriminant function analysis* indicates which variables are most important in accounting for the differences.

In the previous chapter, we mentioned a few times that, if a T^2 or MANOVA is significant, you can use a discriminant function analysis to determine where those differences lie. It's now time to take a look at this technique and see how it can be used (or misused, as is often the case) following these tests or on its own.

Discriminant function analysis (DFA) is used when we have two or more groups, and where each subject is measured on at least two dependent measures. If the groups are different, we would want to know (a) which variables they differ on, and (b) whether they differ more on some variables than on others. The mathematics of the technique derives a function (that is, an equation) which best discriminates between the groups; hence the name. The equation is simply the first variable multiplied by a "weight," plus the second variable multiplied by its "weight," and so on for all of the variables, like this:

$$w_1V_1 + w_2V_2 + \ ... \ + w_pV_p$$

where the w's are the weights and the V's are the variables, for all of the "p" variables. This is like a regression equation, except that we are predicting group membership rather than a particular value of a dependent variable.

One of the best ways to conceptualize what DFA does is to visualize it. We can begin with a relatively simple example of only two groups with two dependent variables. Let's imagine that a researcher wants to see why some post-myocardial infarction patients drop out of an exercise program. She divides her subjects into two groups, compliers and non-compliers, and measures two variables on each person, namely forced expiratory volume (FEV_1), a measure of respiratory function, and an index of "health belief." In the last chapter, we showed how we can summarize the results for the two groups by drawing scatter-plots. We'll do the same thing again, which is shown in Figure 14.1. This time, the two axes are for the variables FEV_1 and health belief, and the two ellipses represent the two groups, compliers and non-compliers.

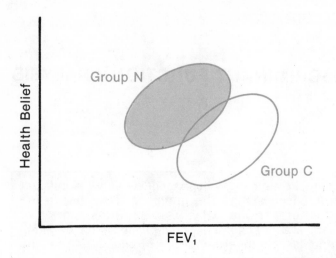

Figure 14.1   Health belief and FEV₁ scores for treatment and control groups

We begin by drawing a line which would best separate these two groups from each other. This is very simple to do by hand: draw a straight line through the two points where the ellipses cross each other, and continue the line a little bit past the point where it crosses one of the axes. This would be Line I in Figure 14.2.

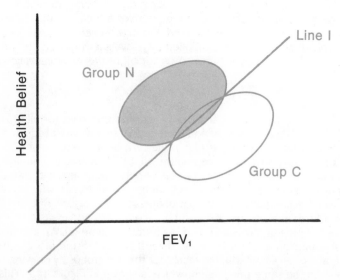

Figure 14.2   Line which best separates treatment and control groups on health belief and FEV₁

Although the two groups fall to either side of this line, it is not the discriminant function. We now draw another line, perpendicular to the first, and passing through the origin; in Figure 14.3, this is Line II. As we'll see in a short while, *this* is the discriminant function line. What we can now do is project each point in the ellipses onto Line II. This will result in two bell curves, one for each ellipse. The maximum point of the bell curve falls exactly under the centroid since this is where most of the points cluster. The further away we get from the centroid, the fewer points there are, so the bell curve tapers off at the ends, as demonstrated in Figure 14.4.

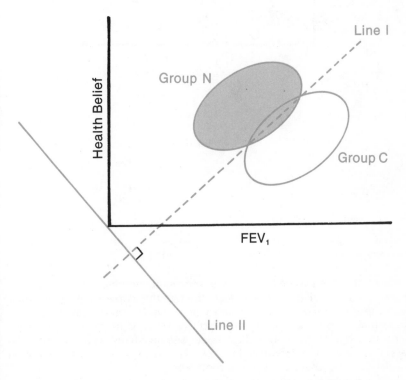

Figure 14.3 Discriminant function between treatment and control groups

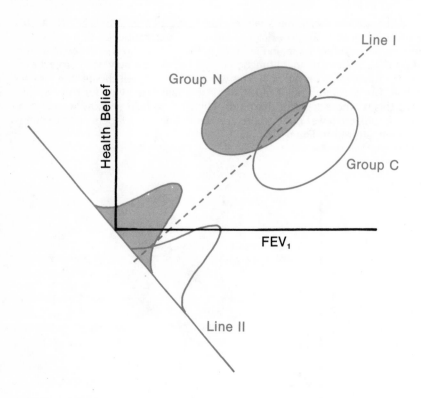

Figure 14.4 Discriminant function showing distributions

Notice that the two bell curves overlap to some degree, corresponding to the overlap in the ellipses. This reflects the fact that some subjects in Group C (compliers) have scores more similar to the Group N (non-compliers) centroid than to their own Group C) centroid, and vice versa. In more concrete terms, some non-compliers have better FEV_1 values and health beliefs than some compliers. The greater the difference between the groups, given the same degree of variability, the less overlap there should be.

First, each subject, rather than being represented by a *pair of points* (his or her scores on the two variables), can now be represented by *one point*, a number along this line. This number is determined by plugging each person's scores on the variables into the equation, which yields a discriminant score. Now for each individual subject, we can see whether his or her scores are more similar to the centroid of the compliance group or the non-compliance group. Since this line is a representation of the person's discriminant score, Line II rather than Line I is referred to as the discriminant function. Second, the point at which the two curves cross, under Line I, minimizes the overlap and results in the smallest number of cases being misclassified.

Let's spend a few minutes discussing the equation itself. As we said before, it includes all of the variables, and each variable is multiplied by a different weight. This should sound familiar to you, since it's the same idea we discussed in relation to a regression equation. If the variables are standardized (i.e., all variables have been transformed to have the same mean—zero—and the same standard deviation—one), then the larger the absolute value of the weight, the more that variable contributes to discriminating between the groups. Weights close to zero indicate variables that don't add much to the discriminating power of the equation. Thus, running a DFA after a significant T^2 or MANOVA can tell us, by examining the discriminant weights, on which variables the groups differ.

What if there are more than two groups? Except in highly unusual cases, one discriminant function won't be sufficient to discriminate among three or more groups. In fact, by the mathematics of DFA, if there are K groups, there will be $K-1$ discriminant functions. The first function is the most "powerful" one, the one which best separates one group from the remaining ones. The second function is best in accounting for the remaining variance and may help in discriminating among the other groups. This pattern continues on down the line, with the last or last few functions (assuming four or more groups) possibly not adding much to our ability to discriminate among the groups.

Statisticians don't like phrases such as "doesn't add too much." Being literal sorts of folks, we want a number whereby we can say either, "Yes, this additional function is useful," or "Forget it." The test for the significance of a discriminant function is called Wilk's lambda test, and is printed out by the various "canned" DFA programs. (Remember from our discussion of lambda with respect to MANOVA that the *smaller* it is, the more significant.) The significance of lambda is tested with a chi-square; if the probability of the chi-square is less than the usual 0.05, then that function contributes to the discriminating power; if it is not significant, it (and all the succeeding functions) can be disregarded.

Also, DFA can be used, and usually is, with more than two variables. Graphing it gets difficult, but the mathematics handles it with relative ease. However, there are two problems in adding more groups and variables. First, the more variables there are, the less stable the solution is, in general. That is, upon replication, the variables which appeared to be powerful discriminators the first time may not be so at later times. This should sound familiar since the same thing was discussed in regression analysis. The second problem is that the more functions there are, the more difficult the interpretation becomes. One function is easy, two you can handle, but trying to understand three or more significant discriminant functions can be likened to deciphering the Rosetta Stone without knowing any Greek. So, as the Bauhaus has taught us, like many things in life, less is more.

In reading articles in which DFA was used, you'll probably run across the term "step-wise," as in "a step-wise solution was used." Just as in regression analysis, a step-wise solution considers variables one at a time. The equation first considers the variable that best discriminates among the groups. Then, a second variable is added, the one that most improves the discriminating ability of the equation. This process of adding one variable at a time is continued until one of two things happens: either all of the variables are entered into the equation, or adding the remaining variables doesn't appreciably (read "statistically significantly") improve the power of the equation in discriminating among the groups.

The advantages and disadvantages of this procedure are similar to those when it's used in regression analysis. On the positive side, it allows you to pick from a large number of variables a smaller subset with almost equal discriminating ability, and ranks the variables in order of their importance. This can be very useful when it's necessary to cut down the number of variables to improve the ratio of subjects to variables, explain group differences most parsimoniously, or replicate the study with a smaller number of tests.

The primary disadvantage is an interpretive one. If two of the variables are correlated, then one may end up in the function but the other may not. The reason for this is that, as with step-wise regression, a variable is entered if it improves the discrimination over and above the effect of the previously entered variables. So, if forced vital capacity (FVC) is highly correlated with FEV_1, and if FEV_1 has already been entered, then FVC may not give us any additional information and won't be part of the final equation. This feature is terrific if we want to select a smaller set of variables for some purpose, but it can lead us down the garden path if we conclude from this that the groups don't differ in terms of FVC. They *do* differ, but FVC doesn't explain any more of the differences than we already know about from their differences on FEV_1.

Unfortunately there is yet one more aspect to DFA; classification analysis. Classification analysis is a separate statistical technique that exists independently from DFA, but the two techniques are most frequently encountered together, so we'll treat them together. Recall that we can use DFA in a number of ways: to indicate on which variables two or more groups differ; to choose a subset of variables which do an equally good job as the original, larger set; and to classify a given subject into a group. We'll look for a moment at the use of DFA for classification.

If we go back to the original figure, each subject's scores can be plugged into the discriminant function and reduced to a single point on Line II. Then, if he or she falls on one side of the cut-off (Line I), then that person can be predicted to be in the compliant group, and on the other side, in the non-compliant group.

This type of analysis can be used in a number of ways. Perhaps the most useful although least used way is to derive a series of equations on one set of groups, and then use those functions to predict where a *new* subject falls. The way classification analysis is *most* used is to check on the "goodness" of the discriminant functions. Here, the same people are used to generate the equations, and then to be "classified," by plugging their original scores back into the functions. If Subject 1 was originally from Group A, and the equations place him closest to the A centroid, then we've got a "hit." However, if the equations say he is more similar to Group B's centroid, then we have a "miss." So, for all subjects, we have two indices of group membership, the *actual* group the person is from, and the group *predicted* on the basis of the equations. From this, we can construct a two-way table, with the rows being the actual group and the columns being the predicted one. Let's make up a simple example, where

Group A has 100 subjects and Group B has 50. The results are shown in Table 14.1.

Table 14.1   Two-way Table to Demonstrate Accuracy of Classification

Actual Group	Predicted Group		
	A	B	Total
A	75	25	100
B	20	30	50
Total	95	55	150

As we can see, 75 of the subjects in Group A are correctly placed using the equation, and 30 of the 50 Group B subjects have been put in the right group. Overall, 70 percent of the subjects have been correctly classified by the discriminant function. Often, a chi-square is calculated on this table to see if these results differ from a chance finding.

Moreover, most of the packaged computer programs for DFA can also tell us how confidently we can place a person in a given group, by assigning a probability level to that person belonging to each of the groups. Thus, for one person, the probabilities that he falls into each of the three groups may be 0.85, 0.09, and 0.06 respectively, and we would be fairly sure of our classification of him into the first group. But, if the probabilities assigned to another person are 0.24, 0.40, and 0.36, we would have to say she most resembles the second group, but we wouldn't be as sure, since there is an almost equal probability that she can be from the last group.

Example 14.1

A researcher studying a group of insomniacs and a group of normal sleepers measures the following variables on each subject: (i) sleep onset latency, (ii) total sleep time, (iii) total REM time, (iv) percent REM, (v) total time in Stages 3 and 4, and (vi) percent time in stages 3 and 4.

Question 1

How many equations will there be?

Answer

Since there are only two groups, there will be just one discriminant function, irrespective of the number of variables.

C.R.A.P. **DETECTOR #14.1**

The researcher should report how "good" the discriminant function(s) is. Is it significant? How well does it classify the subjects? And so forth.

Question 2

What is the minimum number of subjects she should have in each group?

Answer

Since there are 6 dependent variables, she should have at least 60 subjects in each group.

C.R.A.P. **DETECTOR #14.2**

Yet again, the old 10-to-1 rule.

Question 3

A step-wise solution yielded 4 variables: latency, total sleep time, total REM, and total time in stages 3 and 4. From those data she concluded that normals and insomniacs do not differ in the *percentage* of time they spend in REM and deep sleep. Was she right?

Answer

We don't know. Since percent REM and deep sleep are probably correlated with the other variables, it is likely that they didn't enter into the equation because they didn't add any new information. Still, the groups could have differed significantly on these variables.

C.R.A.P. **DETECTOR #14.3**

Be cautious in interpreting the results of a step-wise procedure, especially in determining which variables were *not* entered. Were they really unimportant, or were they simply correlated with other variables that did enter into the equation?

Question 4

She reported that 75 percent of the subjects were correctly classified on the basis of the equation. Can you expect results this good if you now used the equation with your patients?

Answer

No. A discriminant function always does better in "classify-ing" the subjects from which it was derived than with a new group. How much better is extremely difficult to determine.

C.R.A.P. DETECTOR #14.4

The goodness of an equation in classifying subjects should always be tested on a "cross-validation" sample, i.e., a group of new people who were not used in deriving the equation.

FACTOR ANALYSIS
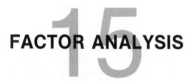

> When many different measures have been taken on the same person, it is possible to determine if some of these tests are actually reflections of a smaller number of underlying factors. Factor analysis explores the interrelationships among the variables to discover these factors.

Perhaps the most widely used (and misused) multivariate statistic is factor analysis. Few statisticians are neutral about this technique. Proponents feel that factor analysis is the greatest invention since the double bed, while its detractors feel it is a useless procedure that can be used to support nearly any desired interpretation of the data. The truth, as is usually the case, lies somewhere in between. Used properly, factor analysis can yield much useful information; when applied blindly without regard for its limitations, it is about as useful and informative as Tarot cards. In particular, factor analysis can be used to explore the data for patterns, confirm our hypotheses, or reduce the many variables to a more manageable number. Before we discuss these uses, though, it will be helpful to probe some of the theory of factor analysis.

CORRELATION AMONG VARIABLES

The basic assumption is that it may be possible to explain the correlation among two or more variables in terms of some underlying "factor." For example, we would not see our inability to run as fast as we did last year, our aches and pains that we feel afterwards, and the nap we have to take to recuperate, as reflecting three unrelated phenomena, but as all reflecting one underlying cause: we are getting older. To take another example, if we see a patient's temperature and white blood count (WBC) both increasing, we would say that these two signs are due to one common cause, namely an infection. In the jargon of statistics, these causes are called factors. Sometimes they refer to observable phenomena, but more often the factors are hypothetical constructs, such as intelligence, depression, or coping ability. We cannot measure intelligence directly, we can only infer its existence from behaviors which we hypothesize are based on it, such as school grades, the time needed to figure out a puzzle, or the accuracy in defining words. Our theory states that all are influenced by this hypothetical thing we call "intelligence." If we test a number of people and find that these three measures are correlated, we would state that they are attributable to an underlying factor of intelligence.

WEIGHING OF SCORES

Factor analysis, then, is a technique which enables us to determine whether the variables we've measured can be explained by a smaller number of factors. Let's assume that, as in the previous example, we've measured or recorded a person's average school grade, the time needed to solve five puzzles, and the score on a vocabulary test. Just on an intuitive basis, we can say that all three scores are related to intelligence. However, we also suspect that intelligence may be more important for one measure than for another. Grade point average, for instance, can be influenced by motivation in school and may not be as "true" a measure of intelligence as vocabulary. We can show this by "weighing" each of the three scores: the higher the weight, the closer that variable is associated with intelligence. Factor analysis of these three scores, which we've measured on a number of people, is demonstrated in Table 15.1.

Table 15.1   Factor Analysis of Intelligence Measures

Variable	Load
Grade point average	$= 0.60 \times F$
Puzzle times	$= 0.75 \times F$
Vocabulary score	$= 0.85 \times F$

where F is the factor. This tells us that the vocabulary score loads highly on the intelligence factor, that puzzle time loads slightly less, and grade point average loads least. These weights are really just correlations: the correlation between vocabulary and the factor is 0.85, while it is 0.75 for puzzles, and 0.60 for grade point average.

FACTOR LOADING

This example is artificial in two respects: There are very few variables, and only one factor was found. Usually we would have many more variables, and will find more factors, but the basic ideas are the same. A more difficult question is: "Are measures of performance in medical school related to these three indices of intelligence?" Suppose that, as part of the admission battery, we gathered data on these measures. Then, after graduation, we recorded each student's medical school grade point average, a rating of performance on an inpatient unit, and one of outpatient clinic performance. To save some room, we'll refer to the variables in the following tables as

X_1 = Pre-med grade point average
X_2 = Puzzle times
X_3 = Vocabulary score
X_4 = Medical school grade point average
X_5 = Inpatient rating
X_6 = Outpatient rating

The data matrix would be too big to show in its entirety, since we would probably be dealing with between 100 and 200 students. The first few lines of the matrix appear in Table 15.2.

Table 15.2   Effect on Performance in Medical School of Intelligence Measures

Subject	Variables					
	X_1	X_2	X_3	X_4	X_5	X_6
1	3.7	158	17	3.9	8.8	9.2
2	3.6	164	19	3.7	9.1	9.0
3	3.8	137	21	3.8	8.5	7.9

Factor analyzing this, our results are tabulated in Table 15.3

Table 15.3   Factor Analysis of Intelligence Measures in Medical Students

Variable	F_1	F_2
X_1	0.60	0.25
X_2	0.75	0.10
X_3	0.85	0.30
X_4	0.50	0.45
X_5	0.15	0.85
X_6	0.10	0.90

A table like this, which will be found every time you do a factor analysis, is called a factor-loading matrix, or factor matrix. Notice that the rows are different from the original data matrix. With the data, each row represented a different subject; here, each row is a different variable. Similarly, the columns refer to factors, not variables as in the data matrix. This table tells us how highly each variable correlates with, or loads on, each factor, just as in the first example. The only difference is that now each variable loads on two factors, rather than only one.

In this example, it appears as if the first factor consists of three variables; X_1, X_2, and X_3, and we could label this factor "intelligence." Two variables, X_5 and X_6, load highly on the second factor, so we can call this factor, "clinical skills." Variable X_4 is a bit more of a problem, since it loads about equally on both factors, and doesn't seem to belong exclusively to either one. Let's digress for a moment and discuss three things: "How did we determine which variables went with each factor?" "How did we name the factor?" "And what determines how many factors we end up with?"

Usually, a variable is assigned to the factor on which it loads most highly. So, since variable X_1 loaded 0.60 with Factor 1 and 0.25 with Factor 2, we would assign it to the first factor. There are times, as with X_4, that a variable loads on two or more factors almost equally. In such cases, it would have to be assigned to all the factors on which it loads highly. You may well ask, "How equal is 'almost equal'?" Based on all of our readings in this area, we can give a definitive answer: "We don't know." This is one of the many areas in statistics where experience and judgment are as important as statistical significance levels. A general rule of thumb, with the emphasis on "general", is that, if one factor loading is within 0.05 of the highest one, consider it equal. With the latest example, since the two factor loadings are 0.50 and 0.45 for variable X_4, we would say that it loads on both factors. The naming of factors is even more arbitrary. Once you've determined which variables load on a factor, you can try to puzzle out what those variables have in common, and assign a name accordingly. Some people feel that this is an exercise only in semantics, and use the unimaginative (if highly useful) names, Factor 1, Factor 2, and so on.

EIGENVALUES

The third issue of how many factors will there be, has both an easy and a hard answer. The easy answer is that the total number of factors will equal the number of variables. However, the number of useful factors will be substantially less. Each factor has associated with it an eigenvalue, which is simply the amount of variance in the data explained by that factor. Owing to the way in which factor analysis is done, the first factor found (or "extracted," in our jargon) has the highest eigenvalue, the next factor has the second highest eigenvalue, and so on down the line. Probably the first few factors will account for the bulk of the variance, and the later ones will account for only a small proportion of it. The rule most commonly used is the so-called "eigenvalue-one" rule: keep only those factors whose eigenvalues are greater than 1.0, and throw out the rest. In the latest example, both of the factors have eigenvalues greater than 1.0 and we have assumed that the other four factors were not listed because their eigenvalues were less than 1.0.

ROTATION OF AXES

At this point, we would have completed the first two steps of a factor analysis; we have extracted the factors, and kept only those factors whose eigenvalues were greater than 1.0. The results of these steps, which are referred to as principal components analysis, is displayed in the factor-loading matrix, as in the previous example. Some people stop at this point, but most researchers take one further step, they rotate the factors. You may wonder why this step is necessary, since the factor-loading matrix tells us what we want to know. Here, we must confess that the numbers in Table 15.3 were not derived from an actual factor analysis; we made them up to illustrate a point. In so doing, the results were much neater than they usually are in real life. Table 15.4 represents a more realistic version of a factor-loading matrix.

Table 15.4   Factor-loading Matrix for Six Variables

Variable	F_1	F_2
X_1	0.45	0.56
X_2	0.56	0.38
X_3	0.40	0.52
X_4	0.55	−0.60
X_5	0.72	−0.10
X_6	0.78	−0.36

Although it may not appear obvious, this table differs from the the previous one in three important respects. (1) As often happens, the first factor is a general factor; most (or all, as in this case) of the items load significantly on it. Sometimes, this in itself is an important finding, but more frequently it is not. It simply may reflect that the fact that all of the measures are taken on the same people introduces a degree of correlation among the measures. In most instances, we would want to eliminate this intra-individual correlation and look only at inter-item relationships. (2) The succeeding factors are often bipolar factors; that is, there are some items with significant positive loadings (e.g., variables X_1 through X_3), and some with significant negative ones (variables X_4 and X_6; the loading for variable X_5 on Factor 2 is too low to worry about). This situation is more difficult to interpret than if all of the values were positive or negative. (3) Some variables load significantly on two or more factors. This is called factorial complexity in our argot. As with factors being bipolar, there is nothing wrong with factorial complexity from a statistical point of view, only that the interpretation of the items and the factors is more difficult.

We can illustrate these three points more clearly by making a graph in which the X axis represents Factor 1 and the Y axis is Factor 2, then plotting the variables. For example, variable X_1 loads 0.45 on Factor 1 and 0.56 on Factor 2, so we put a "1" (to indicate variable 1) 0.45 units along the X axis and 0.56 units up the Y axis. The results for all six variables are shown in Figure 15.1.

We can immediately see three problems. (1) All of the points are well to the right of the origin, indicating that they all load on Factor 1. (2) Some points are above the X axis (where the Y axis is positive), and some are below it (where Y is negative), reflecting the fact that Factor 2 is bipolar. (3) The points fall toward the center of the quadrants, since they load on both factors; they are factorially complex.

ORTHOGONAL ROTATION

We can lessen the effect of these problems with a relatively simple technique. Imagine that the points remain where they are, but rotate the axes clockwise about 40°, keeping them at right angles to each other. Figure 15.2 shows the new axes with a dashed line. The new axis for Factor 1 has been relabeled F_1', and the redrawn F_2 axis is called F_2'.

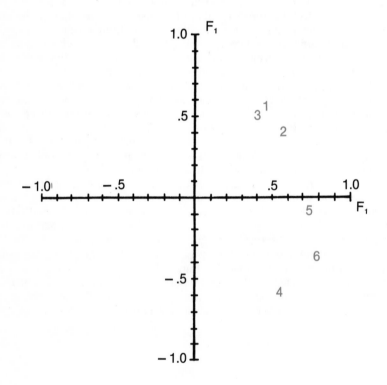

Figure 15.1   Correlations between variables and two factors

Notice that all three problems have been diminished to varying degrees. Three variables (X_1 to X_3) lie quite close to axis F_2', showing that they do not load on the first factor. Second, most of the variables have only positive loadings. The one exception is X_4, which has a negative loading on Factor 2; however, the magnitude is low (-0.15) and probably not significant. Lastly, we have reduced the factorial complexity to a considerable degree. If we had three factors, the same type of rotation would have been done, but in three dimensions rather than two. If we ask the computer to rotate the axes, we would be provided with a rotated factor matrix, which is interpreted in exactly the same way as the original factor matrix.

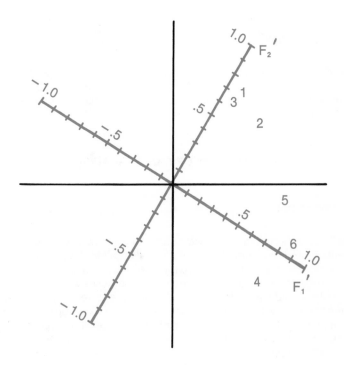

Figure 15.2 Correlation between variables and rotated factors

OBLIQUE ROTATION

Before we leave this topic, it is worthwhile to mention some phrases you may encounter with respect to rotations. In introducing this topic, we said, "rotate the axes ... keeping them at right angles to each other." We refer to this type of rotation as an orthogonal rotation. Once in a while, a researcher may relax this condition and allow the axes to be rotated without preserving the right angles among them. This is called an oblique rotation. Of course, the same data could be analyzed using both methods. What is the difference between orthogonal and oblique? In the former, the factors are totally uncorrelated with one another, while in the latter, the angle between factors reflects their degree of correlation: the closer to 0° and the further from 90°, the higher the correlation. An orthogonal rotation is easier to interpret, which is probably why it is preferred, but an oblique rotation often provides a more accurate reflection of reality.

VARIMAX ROTATION

There are many ways of determining the optimal rotation, and statisticians don't agree among themselves on which is best. However, the most widely used criterion is that the rotation should maximize the variance explained by each factor. Consequently, this technique is call varimax rotation.

APPLICATION OF FACTOR ANALYSIS

Exploration of Data

Finally, let's discuss the three ways factor analysis can be used: exploration, confirmation, and reduction. In exploration (also called data dredging or a fishing expedition by those who object to this use of factor analysis), we begin with a large number of variables but no explicit hypotheses about how they hang together. We would use factor analysis in this case to reveal patterns of interrelationships among the variables that aren't otherwise apparent. For example, we may wish to develop a battery of tests to measure cognitive recovery following a shunt operation for normotensive hydrocephaly. Not knowing beforehand which tests tap similar areas of functioning, we would begin with a large number of them, and then use factor analysis to help us determine which tests cluster together. That is, we may find one set loading on a factor we can call visual motor coordination, another factor of spatial memory, and so on. In this way, we let the analysis indicate patterns within the data.

Confirmation of Hypotheses

We can also use factor analysis to confirm our hypotheses about the data. This application often is made when designing a new test, or replicating an experiment, or testing a theory. In these cases, we hypothesize ahead of time which factors should emerge. For example, let's say we want to develop a paper-and-pencil test to measure knowledge of, and attitudes toward, contraceptive use. We would begin by writing a large pool of items to tap these two areas and trying out the questionnaire on a number of people. If we wrote our questions well, two factors should emerge, one comprised of knowledge-related questions and one of attitude-related questions. If there is a third factor, or if some items load on both factors, it would be a signal that the item is not measuring what we thought it should, and it's back to the drawing boards.

Reduction of Data

In some situations, we may want to reduce the number of variables we have on each subject for later analyses. That is, we may start off with a large number of items per subject, but for various reasons we'll discuss in a moment, want only five or six summary scores on people. Here, we could use each factor as a type of scale. If, say, 12 of the items load significantly on Factor 2, we could simply sum a person's score on those 12 variables and use this total as a new variable, effectively reducing the number of variables by 11. The major reason for this use of factor analysis is often to increase the subject-to-variable ratio, so that in subsequent analyses, the 10:1 rule wouldn't be violated.

Example 15.1

In order to determine which factors affect return to work following coronary bypass surgery, an investigator gives a number of cardiac, pulmonary, and psychological tests to a group of subjects, yielding a total of 35 scores.

Question 1

What is the minimum number of subjects he should have to factor analyze the results?

Answer

If he throws all the tests into one big factor analysis, he should have at least 350 subjects.

Question 2

Is there any way he can get around this, since there are only 50 patients a year in his town who receive the procedure?

Answer

He can factor analyze each set of findings (cardiac, pulmonary, and psychological) independently, and then later deal with the three sets of factors as if they were variables.

Question 3

Not having read this book, he throws all of the variables into the pot at the same time, and reports that he ended up with six factors, with eigenvalues of 4.13, 3.87, 3.29, 2.85, 1.71, and 1.03, respectively. Would you be as ecstatic as he was about his results?

Answer

Definitely not. Since there were 35 variables, the sum of the eigenvalues for all of the factors would be 35. The six factors with eigenvalues greater that one account for only 48 percent of the variance (4.13 + ... 1.03 = 16.88; 16.88/35 = 0.48). That means that 52 percent of the variance among the 35 variables is *not* accounted for by the six factors. Ideally, the retained factors should account for at least 60 percent, and preferably 75 percent, of the variance.

Question 4

He reported only the eigenvalues of the retained factors and the names he assigned to them. What else is missing from the results?

Answer

Since there are so many options to choose among when using factor analysis, he should also have reported (1) the method used to extract the principal components; (2) whether a rotation was done; (3) if so, what type; and (4) the factor loading table itself.

CLUSTER ANALYSIS

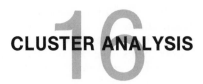

In factor analysis, we determined whether different variables can be grouped together in some specific way. With cluster analysis, we examine whether people (or animals, or diagnoses, or any other entities) can be grouped on the basis of their similarities.

In the previous chapter, we discussed how factor analysis can be used to find interrelationships among variables. In this chapter, we will examine a class of techniques, collectively termed cluster analysis, which attempts to find interrelationships among objects. (Despite objections from humanists and others, people are referred to as "objects," as are animals, psychiatric diagnoses, or geographical areas. This is just jargon, not a philosophical statement.) There are two major (and many minor) classes of cluster analytic techniques, with about a dozen different methods in each class. And the number is still growing. Complicating the issue even further, various authors use completely different names to refer to the same method. We can't begin to mention, much less discuss, all of these different techniques, so refer to some of the books and articles referenced in the Bibliography if you want to plow your way through this field.

METHODS OF CLASSIFYING DATA

Cluster analysis began with the attempts of biologists to classify similar animals and plants into groups and to distinguish them from other groups of animals and plants. For a long time, this was done by the individual taxonomist (that is, someone who classifies, not an agent for the Revenuers) on the basis of his perception of anatomical and morphological similarities and differences. Needless to say, this led to many disputes among taxonomists, since what was obvious similarity to one person was just as obviously a difference to another. In 1963, Sokal and Sneath wrote a book entitled *Principles of Numerical Taxonomy*, which attempted to introduce some mathematical rigor to the field. However, rather than bringing people together (which, after all, is one of the aims of classification), it served to broaden the points of argument and to introduce yet another area of disagreement. Now, people were fighting over the best numerical technique, as well as battling those who maintained that the intuitive process of classification could not be reduced to "mindless" computer algorithms.

So, what is all this debate about? As you may have already deduced, "clustering" and "classifying" are synonymous terms which refer to the grouping of objects into sets on the basis of their similarities, and the differentiating between sets based on their differences. As an example, all clinicians "know" that they can classify their patients on other than diagnostic bases. Those who come in only when they're on death's doorstep; those who make appointments every time a new pimple appears, which they are convinced is the first sign of melanoma; a group which will blindly follow any advice given; another set of patients who won't take their medications, no matter how often they're told to do so; and so on. How would a clinician go about classifying these patients on a less subjective, more objective basis?

Before he can begin, the investigator must decide what he thinks the world is actually like, since this will dictate which of the two major classes of cluster analysis he will use: hierarchical methods or partitioning methods. This choice is a very important one, since analyzing data with the wrong method will most likely yield some results, but they may be quite discrepant from "reality." As the name implies, hierarchical clustering methods end up looking like trees, such as those drawn by zoologists to classify the animals: the kingdom of animals is subdivided into various phyla, which in turn branch into different classes, and so on down the line, until each animal can be uniquely placed within its particular species or subspecies. The underlying assumption is that each subspecies is unique, but that all of the subspecies within a given species have something in common. Similarly, the species are different from each other, but we can move up to a higher level of organization, the genus, in which all of its species are somehow related. So, if our investigator chose this method, it would reflect an implicit or explicit belief that there is a hierarchy of patient types: they can, for example, be subdivided into groups, namely the overusers, the underusers, and the good guys. Each of these groups can be further subdivided and each group may have a different number of subgroups, and so on. At the end, there will be as many little groups as patient types, all arranged in a hierarchical manner.

Partitioning methods, on the other hand, assume that each cluster is different from every other cluster, and there is no higher level of organization that can group the clusters together. Among major diagnostic groupings, the carcinomas form one cluster, quite distinct from the arteriosclerotic diseases, and both of these differ from the hemopoetic disorders. Choice of this method would reflect a "model" of the world where the chronic complaining patients would have nothing in common with the non-compliant ones, who in turn are different from the hypochondriacs.

HIERARCHICAL METHODS

Since it is the easier method to understand, let's begin by discussing the hierarchical method. As a first step, the investigator would record various measures from or about each patient. This may include age, sex, marital status, number of visits in the past 12 months, proportion of visits where nothing was found, index of the severity of illness at each presentation, and anything else deemed relevant. We begin by constructing a matrix, where each entry is an index of similarity between patients. The problem at this point is to decide what we mean by similar or dissimilar.

The earliest similarity index was simply the correlation coefficient where, instead of correlating two variables across all subjects, two subjects were correlated across all variables. You may still run across the terms "Q-type correlation," "Q-type factor analysis," or "inverse factor analysis," which refer to this way of correlating people, and then factor analyzing the matrix. This was the original "cluster analysis." Articles using this term should be at least 20 years old, or the author hasn't kept up with the times. There are many theoretical problems associated with correlating two subjects across variables as an index of similarity. For example, we normally interpret a correlation as meaning, "On the basis of Subject 1's score on Test X, I would predict that his score on Test Y would be ..." This makes sense since X and Y are related and the same person is taking both tests. If we turn this around and correlate across tests, we would have to say that, "On the basis of Subject 1's responses, I would predict that Subject 2 will do ..." However, unlike two tests done by the same person, Subject 1 is independent from Subject 2, so that the logic breaks down completely.

Moreover, the correlation coefficient cannot even tell us if the *pattern* of scores on the various tests is similar from one person to another. Let's take a look at Figure 16.1. In A the two people have parallel profiles, differing only in level. As we would expect, the correlation is +1.0. But, the correlations for B and C are also +1.0, since the scores for one person are related linearly to the other person's scores in each case. For these and many other reasons, the correlation coefficient isn't (or, at least, shouldn't be) used as an index of similarity.

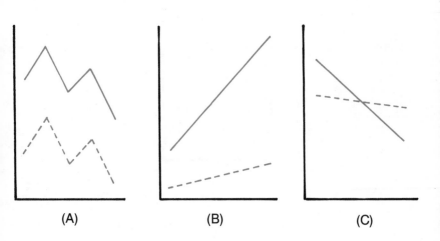

(A)   (B)   (C)

Figure 16.1 Various ways two curves could yield a correlation of +1.0

In its place, similarity is now measured by some index of the *distance* between the sets of points. The difficulty here, as with many multivariate procedures, is an embarrassment of riches. There are probably three dozen different indices, ranging from the simple measurement of the distances between the raw scores called the "unstandardized Euclidian distance" to highly sophisticated techniques with such forbidding names as the "Minkowski metric," "Mahalanobis' D²," or the "city block metric." All of the measures try to do the same thing, to come up with one number that expresses how far apart or how dissimilar two sets of scores are from one another. If one method were clearly superior to all of the others, there would be only one measure around. The plethora of indices indicates that each method has its limitations and that each index makes realistic or tenable assumptions. More unfortunately, the various indices can give rise to quite different solutions.

For the sake of simplicity, assume the investigator collected data from only six patients, whom we'll call A through F. Naturally, by this point, you know enough that *you* would never settle for such a small sample size, especially with so many variables. We start by calculating our 6 x 6 similarity matrix. If we find that B and E have the highest similarity index, we would draw a line connecting them (Figure 16.2). We consider B and E together to be one group and go back to our similarity matrix, which now is of size 5 × 5, to find the next highest index.

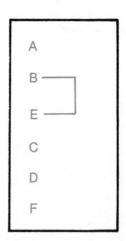

Figure 16.2   Step 1 of the dendogram

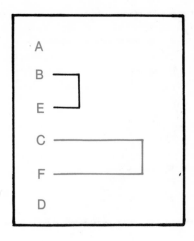

Figure 16.3   Step 2 of the dendogram

We may find that C and F are most similar, and we would draw it as in Figure 16.3. The lines connecting C and F are longer than those connecting B and E because C and F are more dissimilar from each other than B is from E.

In essence, the shorter the horizontal lines, the more similar the objects. We now have four "objects" to group; two objects of one member each (A and D) and two objects which have two members each (BE and CF). If our next highest similarity index reveals that BE is most similar to A, our tree graph or dendogram is portrayed in Figure 16.4.

We continue this process until all of the objects are joined as, for example, in the final dendogram (Figure 16.5).

Thus, the "family" can be divided into two groups, one consisting of patients A, B, and E, and the other comprising of patients C, F, and D. The first group of patients can itself be subdivided into two groups, A and BE, as can the second, into CF and D. Since each step of the process combines the two objects or groups that are most similar, each branch always has two twigs. In real situations, the smallest usable cluster will contain at least five objects. The researcher must decide, almost on a clinical basis, what these objects have in common, and how they differ from the other sets. This is similar to naming factors in factor analysis.

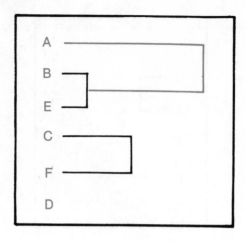

Figure 16.4   Step 3 of the dendogram

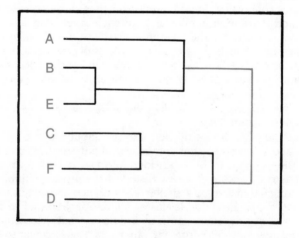

Figure 16.5   Last step of the dendogram

How do we know that one object is similar enough to another object or group to be included with it? There are various criteria with which to work, and again, each criterion may yield a different solution. These methods are analogous to different types of social organizations. One method is like a club that's just forming. The first member, Artie, asks his friend Bob to join. Bob then invites Charlie and David, and so on. Meanwhile, a second, parallel club is being formed in a similar manner, with Stuart asking Tom, who then asks Urquhart (*you* try to think of a name beginning with U) and Victor. This method requires simply that the newcomer be similar to at least one member of the already-existing group. The advantage of this relatively lax criterion is that every person usually ends up in a group. However, we often find that there is a lot of diversity among objects within a group. Object C may join group AB because it is similar to B, and then D may be added because it resembles C, but A and D may be quite dissimilar from one another. This criterion is called single linkage, since the object has to link up with only a single member. It is also referred to as the nearest neighbor, or space contracting method.

We can avoid this problem by being more exclusive, and stipulating that the proposed new member can be blackballed if it differs from *any* of the previous members. This results in a country club atmosphere, where there are nice, tight groupings of almost identical members, but with a lot of outsiders who have little in common with the members or with each other. The term for this criterion is complete linkage, (a.k.a. furthest neighbor, space distorting, and four or five other aliases).

Given these two extremes, it is almost superfluous to say that someone has staked out a middle ground. In this case, it consists of comparing the newcomer with the average of the groups, and joining it to the group whose mean is most similar to its scores, yielding the average linkage, or UPGMC, or nearest centroid method. This is analogous to joining one political group as opposed to another. You join whichever one is most similar to your beliefs, knowing that there will be some degree of heterogeneity of people, who will differ from you to some degree along some dimensions. Despite this diversity, you'd probably be more similar to them than to the people from a different party. Here again, though, we have at least four ways of defining "average," none of which we'll discuss here.

A fourth way is in the tradition of creating as little disturbance as possible. With this approach, an object is joined to the group to which it adds the least within-group variability. That is, it tries out each group in turn, and sticks with the one where its membership increases the variability by the smallest amount. This is the minimum variance criterion, which is also called Ward's method.

Now for a bit of jargon. What we have just described is called an agglomerative hierarchical cluster analysis, since we proceed at each step to join or "agglomerate" two objects or lower-order groups. We can just as easily have gone in the opposite direction, beginning with one large group containing all of the objects, and at each step, dividing it into two parts. This would be called a divisive hierarchical cluster analysis.

PARTITIONING METHODS

As we've mentioned, these procedures assume a specific model of patient taxonomy, namely that there is a hierarchical arrangement of patient types. If the researcher assumed a different model, that each type is unique from all of the others, he would then choose a different brand of cluster analysis,   partitioning method.

Unlike hierarchical methods, the partitioning models do not start off with a similarity matrix. Instead, the investigator makes a set of tentative and somewhat arbitrary clusters. This determination can be made on the basis of intuition, prior knowledge, or, if he feels that there will be six clusters, by stating that the first six objects are the nuclei or seeds of them. The next step is to examine each object and place it in the cluster it most resembles. At this point, most objects have been assigned to one of the groups, and we calculate the centroids of each cluster. Now, each object is compared with each centroid, which means that some of the objects may have to be reassigned to different clusters. This necessitates recomputing the centroids and sifting through all the objects yet again. The process of comparison, assignment, and calculation of centroids is repeated or iterated, until no object needs to be reassigned from one iteration to another.

The various partitioning techniques differ in terms of how the initial clusters are formed, how the final number of clusters are determined, and in the criteria for group membership. We've already discussed the first point briefly, mentioning various options the researcher can choose among. There are also some empirical methods, such as considering that all of the objects belong to one large, heterogeneous group. Then, by some statistical criterion, the group is split into two parts, so that the members of one group are more similar to each other than to the members in the other part. This splitting process is continued until the optimum number of clusters is reached. This may sound a bit like divisive hierarchical clustering, but there is an important difference: There is no assumption that the two "daughter" groups are subsets of the larger group. In partitioning cluster analysis, once a larger group is divided, it ceases to exist as an entity in its own right.

With some forms of partitioning analysis, the investigator must decide at the outset how many clusters will exist at the end, based again on either prior knowledge or sheer guesswork. Other procedures can add or subtract to this initial estimate, depending on the data. If two clusters get too close together, they are merged; if one cluster becomes too heterogeneous, it is split. As usual, religious wars have sprung up over this. On the one hand, the researcher may not know how many groups to expect, so a more empirical criterion is preferred. On the other hand, though, a non-thinking approach can lead to a solution that doesn't make sense on a clinical basis.

Partitioning methods generally use different criteria for group membership than hierarchical methods, but the general principles are the same. The two major points of similarity are: (1) each criterion tries to make the groups homogeneous and different from the other clusters, and (2) each criterion yields dramatically different results.

With so many ways of clustering, computing similarity indices, and determining group membership, it's obviously impossible in one short chapter to go into any depth about the specifics. But, any article which uses cluster analytic techniques should spell out in some detail the exact steps used and *why* those as opposed to some other set of procedures were used. Consequently, our C.R.A.P. Detectors focus on this point.

C.R.A.P. DETECTOR #16.1

Did the authors specify the analytic method used? At the very least, they should state whether they used a hierarchical or a partitioning model, although this may be evident from the results. However, it may not be as readily apparent if they used some other model, or whether an agglomerative or a divisive solution was chosen. The choice of model can produce markedly different results. There should also be some justification for this choice, and why it was preferred, on theoretical grounds, to the other options.

C.R.A.P. DETECTOR #16.2

Was the similarity index specified? Did the authors use a Pearson correlation as their index, followed by a Q-type (or "inverse") factor analysis? This technique has been supplanted by far superior ones over the past two decades, so if the reasons for using it have not been well justified, ignore the study.

C.R.A.P. DETECTOR #16.3

Did they specify the criterion to determine the number of clusters? Again, this may be fixed by the investigator (and if so, why that number of clusters), or determined on statistical grounds. If the latter, which criterion was used?

C.R.A.P. DETECTOR #16.4

Did they state which computer program or algorithm they used? One study found that using exactly the same options with different programs led to different solutions. In order to replicate the results (and see where the other guys went wrong), you should be able to find the program in the computing center or in a specific book.

C.R.A.P. DETECTOR #16.5

Did the authors replicate their results? Since so many results with multivariate procedures don't hold up on replication, don't believe the findings until they have been replicated on a different sample, and preferably by different authors.

CANONICAL CORRELATION

17

> Canonical correlation is an extension of multiple regression. Instead of many predictor variables and one dependent variable, there are now multiple dependent variables.

Up to this point, we've dealt with two classes of correlational statistics: one in which we have just two variables (Pearson's r for interval and ratio data, and Spearman's rho, Kendall's tau and a few others for ordinal data), and a second in which we have a number of independent variables and one dependent variable (multiple regression). There are situations, though, where we would like to explore the interrelationship between two sets of variables.

One major problem faced by all medical schools is trying to predict who of all the applicants would make the best physicians 4 years down the road. The admissions committee looks at a variety of pre-admission variables, such as university grade point average (GPA), MCAT scores, letters of reference, and so on. Let's assume that a school is reevaluating its procedures, and so it decides to wait a few years, and see how these factors relate to the end product. Since the committee has some degree of sophistication, it knows that being a good doctor demands more than just knowledge; it also requires clinical skills. Now let's take a leap of faith and assume that the school can actually measure these two attributes with some degree of accuracy. What can the committee members do with all the data it collects?

There are a number of options open. For example, it can compute two multiple regression equations, regressing the pre-admission variables against each of the outcomes separately. However, this approach assumes that the outcomes are totally independent of each other, and we can safely assume that they're not. The equations will be correct, but it will be difficult to determine the correct probability levels of the statistical tests associated with them. Another alternative would be to combine the two outcome scores into one global measure of performance. This approach has two drawbacks of its own. First, it ignores the pattern of response in that a person high on Knowledge and low on Clinical Skills might have the same global score as a person with the opposite characteristics. The relationship between the two variables may be important, but will be missed with this method. Second, it assumes that Knowledge and Skills have equal weights (that is, are assumed to be equally important), which may be an unduly limiting restriction.

A third method would be to find the best "weights" for the pre-admission scores, and the best weights for the outcomes which would maximize the correlation between the two sets of variables. This is the approach taken in canonical correlation, which we'll examine in this chapter.

As we've said, canonical correlation can be thought of as an extension of multiple linear regression, but where we are predicting to two or more variables, instead of just to one. In fact, we can even ignore the distinction between "dependent" and "independent" variables, and think of canonical correlation as a method of exploring the relationship between two sets of variables. Either set can be called the "predictors," and the other the "criteria," or we can do away with these labels entirely. For example, Set 1 can consist of scores on a test battery at time 1, and Set 2 can comprise scores from the same test administered at a later time. This would be the multivariate analogue of test-retest reliability, where our interest is not in prediction, but in the temporal stability of results. In a different situation, we may gather a number of measures regarding the physical status of cancer patients and a second set of scores on their psychological status. Again, our concern is not in predicting physical status from mental status, or vice versa, but rather in seeing if any relationship exists between these two sets of scores.

CANONICAL VARIATES AND VARIABLES

Let's review what we have so far. Our researcher has gathered two sets of variables; Set A consisting of three pre-admission scores, and Set B of two performance indices. The first step in canonical correlation would be to derive two canonical variates, one for each set of scores. These are not some sort of religious heretics, but are simply summary scores based on the variables in each set. For example, if x_1 is the score for GPA, x_2 the MCAT score, and x_3 the score for the letters of reference, then

$$x_A = B_1x_1 + B_2x_2 + B_3x_3$$

Put into English, the canonical variate for Set A (which we've designated x_A) is derived by multiplying each variable by some "beta-weight."

In a similar manner, we compute a canonical variate for the variables in Set B (consisting of variables x_5 and x_6), and which we'll call x_B. Just to reinforce some of the jargon terms we'll be using later, variables refer to our original measures (GPA, MCAT, and so on); while variates refer to our derived scores, based on multiplying each variable by some weighting factor. The two sets of beta-weights (one for Set A and one for Set B) are chosen to maximize the correlation between x_A and x_B. How this is done is beyond the scope of this book; suffice it to say that no other combination of weights will yield a higher correlation.

PARTIAL CORRELATION

The beta-weights are, in essence, partial correlations. We'll briefly review what this means, since it has major implications for what follows. If we have two predictor variables, say age (A) and serum cholesterol (B), and one criterion variable, such as degree of stenosis (Y), then we can compute simple, run-of-the-mill correlations between each of the predictors and the criterion. Let's make up some figures, and assume r_{AY} is 0.75 and r_{BY} is 0.70. But, we know that age and cholesterol are themselves correlated, say at the 0.65 level. Then, the partial correlation between B and Y is the correlation after *removing the contribution of age* to both cholesterol and stenosis. In this case, the figure drops from 0.70 to 0.42.

So, the beta-weight for variable x_1 is the correlation between x_1 and x_A, eliminating the effects of x_2 and x_3; the beta-weight for x_2 eliminates x_1 and x_3, and so forth.

What this means for canonical correlation is that the two canonical variates that we've derived, x_A and x_B, do not account for all of the variance since only that portion of the variance *uncorrelated with the other variables in the set* was used. We can extract another pair of canonical variates which accounts for at least some of the remaining variability. How many pairs of equations can we get? If we have *n* variables in Set A and *m* variables in Set B, then the number of canonical correlations is the smaller of the two numbers. In our example, *n* is 3 and *m* is 2, so there will be two canonical correlations, or two pairs of canonical variates, x_{A1} paired with x_{B1}, and x_{A2} paired with x_{B2}.

These variates are, in some ways, similar to the factors in factor analysis. They are extracted in order, so that the first one accounts for more of the variance than the second, the second more than the third (if we had a third one), and so on. Second, they are uncorrelated with each other ("orthogonal," to use the jargon). Third, not all of them need be statistically significant. We usually hope that at least the first one is, but we may reach a point where one pair of variates, and all of the succeeding ones, may not be. There is a statistical test, based on the chi-square, which can tell us how many of the correlations are, in fact, significant.

REDUNDANCY

So, what we need at this point are two types of significance tests. First, we have to check how many (if any) of the canonical correlations are significant. As we already mentioned, this is done by a chi-square test developed by Bartlett. Second, if at least one correlation (R_c) is significant, then we have to see if the variables in one set account for a significant proportion of the variance in the other set's variables.

One measure of this is called redundancy, which tries to do for canonical correlation what r^2 does for the Pearson correlation. However, unlike r^2, redundancy is not symmetrical. That is, if r^2 is 0.39, then 39 percent of the variance of variable X can be explained by variable Y, and 39 percent of the variance of Y can be accounted for by X. But, in the multivariate case, Set A may account for 50 percent of the variance in the Set B variables, but Set B may account for only 30 percent of the Set A variance. The figures for redundancy are always less than the square of R_c; they are often much less and may, indeed, be as low as 10 percent even if the magnitude of R_c is quite respectable.

STATISTICAL SIGNIFICANCE

For our original example, the first table that we would see from a computer print out would look something like Table 17.1. The table is not really as formidable as it first appears. The eigenvalue is simply the square of the canonical correlation and is interpreted in the same way as R^2 in multiple regression: The first set of canonical variates shares 73 percent of their variance, and the second set shares 55 percent. Lambda is a measure of the significance of the correlation and, as always, the smaller values are more significant. Through a bit of statistical hand-waving, lambda is transformed into Bartlett's chi-square which humans (i.e., non-statisticians) find easier to interpret. This table tells us that both equations are statistically significant.

Table 17.1

Number	Eigenvalue	Canonical Correlation	Wilk's Lambda	Chi-Square	D.F.	Significance
1	0.732	0.856	0.121	202.953	6	<0.001
2	0.549	0.741	0.451	76.450	2	<0.001

Having found at least one equation significant, the next step is to figure out the pattern of the variables. What we would then look for in a computer print out would resemble Table 17.2. Notice that this simulated output labels the variables V1 through V5; others may use Xs or the variable names.

Table 17.2

	Set 1			Set 2	
	V1	V2	V3	V4	V5
Equation 1	0.803	0.657	0.260	0.960	0.259
Equation 2	−0.115	−0.182	0.966	−0.279	0.966

We would interpret this as meaning that there are two patterns of responding. People who have high GPAs (V1) and high MCAT scores (V2) do well on knowledge-based criteria (V4). Students who did well in clinical skills (V5) were those with good letters of reference (V3). Most of the time the results are not nearly as clear-cut, but the general principles remain the same.

Although the canonical correlations and eigenvalues were quite high, we cannot assume that redundancy is also high. Actually, there are four redundancies here: how much of the variance the Set 1 variables explain of Set 2 for Equation 1 (r_{11}); the same for Equation 2 (r_{12}); and how much the Set 2 variables explain of Set 1 for Equations 1 (r_{21}) and 2 (r_{22}).

The calculations are really quite simple, being the sum of the squares of each coefficient divided by the number of coefficients, times the eigenvalue. For r_{11}, this would be:

$$[(0.803)^2 + (0.657)^2 + (0.260)^2]/N \times 0.732 = 0.279$$

Just for the sake of completeness, $r_{12} = 0.362$, $r_{21} = 0.179$, and $r_{22} = 0.278$. These, then, tell a somewhat different story, with much of the variance awaiting to be explained.

C.R.A.P. DETECTOR #17.1

What was the ratio of subjects to variables? This issue rears its ugly head yet again. As before, there should be at least 10 subjects for each variable, and some authors recommend a 30 to 1 ratio. Even if we split the difference, then we can ignore most articles, since they don't come even close to a 20:1 ratio.

C.R.A.P. DETECTOR #17.2

Are the R_c values significant? If this important statistic was not mentioned, read no further. However, as we've discussed, don't let the reporters get away with reporting *only* the significance level of R_c, there's more yet to come.

C.R.A.P. DETECTOR #17.3

Do they report redundancy? Actually, they need not report redundancy per se, but there should be some estimate of the variance in one set attributable to the other set. The actual statistic may be a predictive one, or some other one, but somewhere it must be mentioned.

C.R.A.P. DETECTOR #17.4

Was the study cross-validated? As we've said before, multivariate statistics always look good on the original sample. However, don't trust the results unless they've been cross-validated on a new sample or on a hold-out sample (that is, deriving the equations on about 75 percent of the original sample and testing its "goodness" on the remaining 25 percent).

RESEARCH DESIGNS

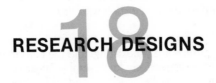

RESEARCH DESIGNS

As we mentioned in the last chapter, statistical methods are excellent for dealing with random variation, but not too useful for eliminating bias in experiments, which must be approached by using appropriate experimental designs. Below is a description of several of the more common ones. Many others exist, and those who are interested should consult one or more of the books listed in the Bibliography.

1. The Randomized Control Trial (RCT)

The RCT provides the strongest research design. A group of people are *randomly* allocated by the researcher to two or more groups. The experimental group receives the new treatment, whereas the control group gets nothing, conventional therapy, or a placebo. For example, our psoriasis patients would be split into two groups by the flip of a coin. The "heads" group would receive clam juice, and the "tails" would receive a placebo concoction. Ideally, in order to minimize various biases, neither the patient nor the researcher knows who got what until the trial is over. This is called "double blind." (If the pharmacist who dispensed the stuff loses the code, it can be called either a "triple blind" or a disaster. In either case, the pharmacist's life is in jeopardy.) More than two groups can be used in an RCT as long as subjects are allocated using some randomizing device.

The major advantage of the RCT is that it ensures that there are no systematic differences between the groups. Since they originally are drawn at random from the same population, randomization ensures that they will be identical except for differences that might arise from chance. In fact, the basis of many statistical tests of hypotheses is that the groups are drawn at random from a population.

However, there are two major drawbacks to the RCT. The first is the cost. Some of the trials designed to look at the effect of aspirin on reinfarction rate cost between three and seven *million* dollars, and the most expensive one of all (at least until now) designed to look at lipids and infarction costs $150 million! Second, patients who volunteer to participate in an RCT, and who agree that the management of their disease be decided by the flip of a coin, may not be representative of patients in general.

2. The Cohort Study

One alternative to the RCT is the cohort study. Two groups (or ''cohorts'') of subjects are identified, one of which, by choice, luck, or chance, has been exposed to the clinical intervention or a putative causal agent, and another which has not. Our researcher, for example, can try to locate a group of clam-juice drinkers and to compare the proportion who have psoriasis with that in a group of abstainers.

Although good cohort studies are not cheap, they are often less expensive than RCTs since the groups are preexisting, and the elaborate safeguards necessary to follow patients prospectively for several years are unnecessary. However, their primary advantages may be feasibility and ethics. If we're studying a helpful intervention, it has not been withheld from those who want it or given to those who don't. Further, it is patently unethical to deliberately expose people to a potentially harmful agent (i.e., such as tobacco smoke or asbestos fibers) so research on health risks must inevitably use this approach. In a cohort study, we locate a group of people who have chosen to smoke or who have been in contact with the putative cause owing to their work, place of residence, travel, or whatever, and thereby avoid these ethical issues.

The major disadvantage is that it is impossible to be sure that the groups are comparable in terms of other factors that may influence the results. Smoking, for example, is related to social class, and jobs that involve exposure to carcinogens are usually related to social class as well. So if smokers have a higher incidence of lung cancer than non-smokers, is it attributable to smoking, social class, occupational exposure, or something else? Even with carefully selected controls, we can never be sure. A second drawback is that, if a certain treatment has become popular for a disorder (e.g., anxiolytics for phobias), it may be hard to find untreated controls. Third, it is difficult, if not impossible, to maintain blindness, at least in the subjects.

3. The Prospective Survey

The prospective survey is similar to the cohort study, but only one group is chosen initially. Some of the subjects will become exposed to the intervention or putative causal agent over time, and others will not. Therefore the outcomes can be looked at in these naturally-occurring groups some time down the road.

The advantages and disadvantages are similar to those of the cohort study. In addition, though, there are some other disadvantages; the primary one being that, at the end, there may be too few subjects in one group to allow for proper analyses.

4. The Case-control Study

In this design, a group of people who already have the outcome (cases) is matched with a group who do not (controls), and the researcher determines the proportion in each who had previously been exposed to the suspected causal factor. For instance in one study the use of exogenous estrogens was compared in one group of women with endometrial cancer to a disease-free control group. The researchers found that more of the cancer patients reported using the hormone than did the other group. However, the weakness of this method was pointed out by a later study, which took as its starting point the supposition that estrogens do not cause cancer, but do lead to bleeding. These women come to the attention of physicians, who then do a biopsy to discover the cause, and find cancer. Women who don't have bleeding may have the same incidence of endometrial cancer, but since no biopsy was done, they were never diagnosed. When using controls to account for this, these researchers found a much lower risk of cancer attributable to estrogens. Because the design is retrospective, it cannot account for other factors that could lead to the outcome. However, in circumstances where the outcome is rare or the time from exposure to outcome is long, this may be the only feasible approach. For example, in most studies of occupational risks related to cancer, in which relatively few people actually go on to develop this disease, delays of 10 to 20 years may be involved, and case-control designs are used.

5. The Cross-sectional Survey

An even weaker method of establishing causal relationships than the prospective survey or the case-control study, is the cross-sectional design, which also uses one group. At one point in time, the subjects are interviewed and/or examined to determine whether or not they were exposed to the agent and whether they have the outcome of interest. For example, a large group of women could be interviewed to determine (a) if they had given birth to a child with a cleft lip and (b) if they had used tricyclics during the pregnancy. If a higher proportion of women who had used these medications had children with this deformity, it may indicate that the antidepressant was responsible.

Cross-sectional surveys are relatively cheap, and subjects are neither deliberately exposed to possibly harmful agents nor do they have treatments withheld from, or imposed on, them. However, in addition to all the problems of prospective surveys, cross-sectional designs have another major one—it may not be possible to state what is cause and what is effect. Schizophrenics, for instance, have larger cerebral ventricles than non-schizophrenics, thus raising the question whether the enlarged ventricles are responsible for the schizophrenia or a result of it? (In fact, they may be caused by the neuroleptic medication.)

6. The Before-after Design

Here, the outcome is assessed prior to, and following, some intervention in one group of subjects. Although common, this design is also weak as the change may be attributable to some other factor. For example, the fact that a group of nursing students score higher on a multiple-choice test after a course in geriatrics than before does not allow the teacher to take credit for their increased knowledge. They may have had an elective at a nursing home or a visit to Grandma's house, or they may have benefitted from taking the exam the first time. Worse still, differences based on a single measure, before and after, may not reflect any intervention at all—just maturation over time.

To some degree these problems can be dealt with by taking multiple measures as described in the chapter, *Time Series Analysis*, but the possibility that something else happened coincident in time with the treatment cannot be excluded.

IMPLICATIONS FOR STATISTICS

What do all these different designs (and there are many others we haven't touched on) have to do with statistics? At the same time, both quite a bit and not too much. For the most part, the decision to use either one statistical test or another depends on the measure more than the design. The results of an RCT can be analyzed with a chi-square or a similar test, if the outcome of interest were nominal or ordinal, such as death or degree of functional improvement measured on a three-point scale. By the same token, t-tests or ANOVAs could be used for continuous outcomes like blood pressure; Hotelling's T^2 or MANOVA for multiple dependent measures; life table analyses for length of survival, and so on. Similarly, the outcome of a prospective or case-control study could be looked at by comparing the proportion of survivors and nonsurvivors in various groups; or by correlating the amount of the outcome (such as a measure of lung functioning) with some other factor (number of cigarettes smoked or length of time at a smelter). So the choice of statistical test is not really related to the experimental design.

However, the statistical tests of significance are predicated on the supposition that the samples were drawn at random from the population. This assumption is violated to a greater or lesser degree in most designs other than the RCT so that the results have to be interpreted with some caution in other designs, both in terms of the actual significance level and in terms of inferring that the results are attributable to the experimental variable and not something else.

ANNOTATED BIBLIOGRAPHY

GENERAL REFERENCES

1. Andrews FM, et al. A guide for selecting statistical techniques for analyzing social science data. Ann Arbor, Michigan: Institute for Social Research, 1974.

   This is a collection of flow charts which guide you in selecting the correct statistics for your data. You begin with the number of variables you have and their scale of measurement. Then you follow the appropriate branches of the decision trees until you find the test you need. An invaluable aid.

2. Bruning JL, Kintz BL. Computational handbook of statistics (2nd ed.). Glenview, Illinois: Scott, Foresman & Co., 1977.

   Once you've found the correct (univariate) test to use, this book will show you how to do it. It uses no theory, no equations, and a minimum discussion of underlying assumptions. In their place, there are step by step procedures for calculating most of the parametric and non-parametric tests you'll ever need. Keep this book chained to your desk. We've already had three copies permanently borrowed.

3. Huff D. How to lie with statistics. New York: WW Norton, 1954.

   This delightful little book focusses entirely on descriptive statistics and illustrates myriad ways in which researchers can distort data to support their conclusions.

4. Castle W N. Statistics in operation. Edinburgh, Churchill-Livingstone.

   This book is worth reading just for the uniquely British humor. Beyond the delightful prose is a nice explanation of basic statistical tests, in a bit more detail than provided here.

PARAMETRIC STATISTICS

There are a number of good introductory books to statistical theory and techniques. Our favorites are:

1. Ferguson GA. Statistical analysis in psychology and education (2nd ed.). New York: McGraw-Hill, 1966.

2. Edwards AL. Experimental design in psychological research (3rd ed.). New York: Holt, Rinehart & Winston, 1968.

3. Loftus GR, Loftus EF. The essence of statistics. Monterey, CA: Brooks/Cole, 1982.

   Far and away the most readable advanced textbook for doers of parametric statistics that we've seen. Covers everything, in an easy and understandable style.

4. Cook TD, Campbell DT. Quasi-experiments: interrupted time-series designs. In: Cook TD, Campbell DT, eds. Quasi-experimentation: design and analysis issues for field settings. Chicago: Rand McNally, 1979.

   An excellent introduction to TSA, presented on an intuitive level without any mathematics.

5. McCain LJ, McCleary R. The statistical analysis of the simple interrupted time-series quasi-experiment. In Cook TD, Campbell DT, eds. Quasi-experimentation: design and analysis issues for field settings. Chicago: Rand McNally, 1979.

   This chapter provides the statistical and theoretical background for the previous article. For those who want it, this is a good place to begin. If you've had an introductory statistics course, or remember your college algebra, this shouldn't be too formidable.

NON-PARAMETRIC STATISTICS

1. Siegel S. Non-parametric statistics for the behavioral sciences. New York: McGraw-Hill, 1956.

   Probably the "bible" of the non-parametric world. The first, and probably still the most readable, introduction to the what, why, and how of non-parametrics.

MULTIVARIATE STATISTICS

Hotelling's T² and MANOVA

We haven't been able to find a good, non-technical introduction. For those who know a bit of matrix algebra (or are willing to learn it from the back of this pamphlet), the best introduction is:

1. Tatsuoka MM. Significance tests: univariate and multivariate. Champaign, Illinois: Institute for Personality and Ability Testing, 1971.

Discriminant Function Analysis

1. Nie NH, et al. Statistical package for the social sciences (2nd ed.). New York: McGraw-Hill, 1975.

   Although written as a manual for the SPSS computer package, there is a very nice, brief introduction to the technique.

2. Tatsuoka MM. Discriminant analysis: the study of group differences. Champaign, Illinois: Institute for Personality and Ability Testing, 1970.

   Again, you'll need some matrix algebra.

Factor Analysis

1. Weiss DJ. Factor analysis and counselling research. J Counsel Psychol, 1970; 17:477-485.

2. Weiss DJ. Further considerations in applications of factor analysis. J Counsel Psychol, 1971; 18:85-92.

   Don't be misled by the titles or the journals; these articles are good, non-technical introductions with wide applicability.

Cluster Analysis

1. Blashfield RK, Aldenderfer MS. The literature on cluster analysis. Multivariate Behavioral Research, 1978; 13:271-295.

   A good guide to the literature. It also provides a translation of the jargon, and a listing of equivalent terms.

2. Blashfield RK. Propositions regarding the use of cluster analysis in clinical research. J Consul and Clin Psychol, 1980; 48:456-459.

This article is an expansion of the C.R.A.P. Detectors, which are actually a summation of this article. Any article by Blashfield on cluster analysis is well worth reading, and written on a level that the intelligent layperson can understand.

3. Borgen FH, Weiss DJ. Cluster analysis and counseling research. J Counsel Psychol, 1971; 18:583-591.

A nice introduction addressed to the clinician with little background in statistics.

Canonical Correlation

1. Weiss DJ. Canonical correlation analysis in counseling psychology research. J Counsel Psychol, 1972; 19:241-252.

Another in the series by Weiss. As is the case for the others, it is well written, clear, and non-technical.

2. Wood DA, Erskine JA. Strategies in canonical correlation with application to behavioral data. Educ Psychol Measur, 1976; 36:861-878.

This article tells you what to look for in evaluating someone else's canonical correlation and gives a good example of how the researcher (and the reader) can be misled if attention isn't given to the C.R.A.P. Detectors.

Research Design

1. Kleinbaum DG, Kupper LL, Morgenstern H. Epidemiologic research. Belmont CA: Lifetime Learning Publications, 1982.

This book will probably tell you more about epidemiology than you really want to know. However, chapters two through five provide an excellent overview of research techniques and designs.

2. Cook TD, Campbell DT. Quasi-experimentation: design and analysis issues for field settings. Chicago: Rand McNally, 1979.

This is the bible of non-experimental research designs and indispensible for the researcher studying phenomena that cannot be subjected to randomized controlled trials.

UNABASHED GLOSSARY

In keeping with the spirit of this book, we have compiled this glossary of various arcane statistical terms, with which you can amaze and impress your friends and colleagues.

Alpha-coefficient: Equivalent of an Italian sports car
Anova: One egg
Autoregression: Thumbsucking in the family car

Bimodal: AC/DC
Biserial correlation: Relationship between Wheaties and Rice Crispies

Cohen's kappa: Rabbi's yarmulka
Construct Validity: Building inspector
Content Validity: Seeing if the test developer is happy
Cross-over design: Christian architecture
Cutting score: Twenty butchers, or music for the Saber Dance

Discriminant function: Opposite of **datcriminant** function
Double-blind trial: First date in a black-out

Goodness-of-fit: Used only in the finest clothing stores

Hotelling's T^2: Device to help architects design inns

Incomplete block: Half-finished apartment building

Kolmogorov-Smirnoff test: Assay for the purity of vodka
Kurtosis: What's at the end of a mangy dog's footsis

Latin square: Roman in conservative garb

Mann-Whitney test: Determination whether a cotton gin were transported across state lines for immoral purposes
Manova: Missionary position
Mean deviate: Misguided sadist
Minimax: Dress for ambivalent women
Multiple regression: Thumbsucking-a-trois

Non-reproducibility: A hysterectomy or vasectomy

Ordinal scale: Device for taking weights in the Vatican
Orthogonal: Birth control pill for males

Paradigms: 20 cents
Poisson distribution: Fishy data from France
Post-test: Intermediate exam for equestrians, falling between a **walk test** and a **canter test**
Profile: A long line of supporters

Rank correlation: Stinkingly low
Raw scores: Data before being cooked by statisticians
Regression toward the mean: Reverting to a sadistic stage of development

Serial dependency: Hooked on Rice Crispies
Simple regression: Ordinary thumbsucking
Square deviate: Transvestite in traditional drag
Standard deviate: Run-of-the-mill homosexual
Stanine: "Hang ten" after the amputation of one toe
Step-wise regression: Thumbsucking in a street-smart kid

T-test: Admission procedure used in English public schools
Type I error: Making one misteak
Type II error: Making two misteakz

INDEX

The letter f following a page number indicates a figure; the letter t following a page number indicates a table.

A

Advanced non-parametric methods, 103–113
    C.R.A.P. detector, 113
    logistic regression, 110–111
    log-linear analysis, 111–112
    Mantel-Haenzel chi-square, 103–105
Alpha errors, 31–34, 32f
Analysis of covariance (ANCOVA), 65–70
    C.R.A.P. detector, 69–70
    sources of variance, 67, 67f
Analysis of variance (ANOVA), 47–55, 49t
    C.R.A.P. detector, 55
    factorial, 51–55
    one-way, 49
        graphical interpretation of, 50f
        Kruskal-Wallis, 86–87
Association, non-parametric measures of, 93–101
Autocorrelation, 75–76
Autoregression model, 76
Autoregressive integrated moving averages (ARIMA) technique, 75
Average deviation, 24

B

Bell-shaped distribution, of data, 25
Beta errors, 31–34, 32f
Beta weights, 53, 154
"Bimodal" distribution, of data, 23, 23f
Binomial test, 81

C

Canonical correlation, 153–157
    canonical variates and variables, 154
    C.R.A.P. detector, 157
    partial correlation, 155
    redundancy, 155–156
    statistical significance, 156–157, 156t
Chi-square, 80–81
    calculation of, 83
    Mantel-Haenzel, 103–105, 104t
        life table analysis, 106–109, 107f–109f, 108t
Classification analysis, 128–129, 129t
Cluster analysis
    C.R.A.P. detector, 151–152

methods of classifying data, 143–151
    hierarchical, 144–149, 145f–148f
    partitioning, 150–151
Coefficient of concordance (Kendall's W), 98–100
Cohen's Kappa, 96–97
Cold remedy study
    ANOVA table for, 54t
    experimental design for, 52t
    graph of interactions, 53f
    using factorial ANOVA, 51–55
Confirmation of hypotheses, 141
Contingency coefficient, 94–95
Continuous variables, 20
Covariance, analysis of (ANCOVA), 65–70
Covariate, 67, 67f
C.R.A.P. detector, 18, 38–39, 45, 55, 62–63, 69–70, 76–77, 91–92, 100–101, 113, 121–122, 129–131, 141–142, 151–152, 157

D

Data
    describing, 19–25
    exploration of, 140
    frequency and distributions, 20–21, 20f, 21f
    means, medians, and modes, 21–23, 22f, 23f
    measures of variation, 23–24
    nominal, tests for, 79–83
    normal distribution of, 24–25, 25f
    process of analyzing, 19
    reduction of, 141
"Data base," 20
"Data set," 20
Dependent variable, definition of, 16
Descriptive statistics, variables and, 15–25
Deviation
    average, 24
    standard, 24
Discrete variables, 20
Discriminant function analysis (DFA), 123–131
    advantages and disadvantages of, 128